KIDS, DRUGS, AND SEX:

PREVENTING TROUBLE

Linda M. Grossman, Ph.D.
and
Deborah Kowal, M.A.

CONTENTS

EXERCISES

Exercises

1

A LOOK AT THE PROBLEM

Teenagers, drugs, and sex are the subject of headlines, law enforcement dilemmas, and hand-wringing episodes for parents. Statistics paint a discouraging picture:

More than 90% of high school seniors have tried alcohol; more than 40% have had five or more drinks in the past two weeks.

Two-thirds (66%) of seniors have tried illicit drugs (mostly marijuana).

Twenty percent of teens have had intercourse before the age of 15; more than 50% have had intercourse by the age of 17.

More than 30% of girls will get pregnant before they outgrow their teen years.

In this chapter we will look beyond these statistics and discuss the who, what, where, when, and why of teen involvement with drugs and sex.

Who?

Certain teens are more likely than others to experiment with drugs and sex. The greatest predictors of whether a teen will try these behaviors (or nearly any other behavior for that matter) are the behaviors of peers and parents. If a teen's friends take drugs or engage in sex, then the teenager will more than likely see that behavior as acceptable. In the same manner, if a parent abuses alcohol or is indiscrete with personal affairs, then the child may assume that these behaviors are acceptable.

We often picture the teen drug user as a loser or a criminal, or the sexually active adolescent as immoral. In reality, many "normal" teenagers experiment with adult behaviors. Although we may find it painful to think our young son or daughter may try drugs, alcohol, or sex, we must still try to maintain a perspective on the matter. First, the experimenting young person is not necessarily defiled and lost to hope. Second, experimentation is not a sure road to regular use or activity.

As a parent, you can make two mistakes when you consider whether your child may some day try drugs or sex. If you find yourself saying "My John (or Jane) would never do that," you are practicing blind denial—a dangerous oversight. Likewise, if you point the finger at your child, certain that he or she will probably get into trouble, you may be declaring guilt on an innocent victim and possibly casting the die.

Why?

"Where have we failed?" is generally the anguished question asked by parents of teens in trouble. Most of the time, that question is an unfair indictment of parents. The reasons teens use drugs or engage in sex can be as complex and wide-ranging as the reasons any of us hold for making decisions about important lifestyle behaviors.

Adolescents are eager to begin trying what they perceive to be adult behaviors. Depending on how these adolescents view the world around them—parents, neighbors, media images—drugs and sex may be tempting adult behaviors. In the same vein, teens may see these behaviors as a way of rebelling against the control of their parents.

Wanting to be more adult and to loosen some of the parental grip is very natural in the development of adolescents as they strive to become more independent human beings. Teens choose certain behaviors for the same reasons many adults do—excitement, the thrill of taking a risk, or the belief that an activity will create pleasure.

On the other hand, some adolescents take drugs or have sex to fulfill certain needs. The abuser of drugs or sex is often a teen who has few friends and who may not have strong support from his family. An intense need to fit in and "be like everyone else" can push some youngsters into doing things they would not otherwise consider. Other youngsters may use drugs or sex to cope with a sense of isolation from peers or family. Sometimes, the young person is just fulfilling a role placed upon him or her as a child: "John is the black sheep of the family." "If anyone will get in trouble, it will be Jane."

A common reason for using drugs or engaging in unintended sex stems from the teen not being prepared to cope with the forces that may influence him or her. For example, many teens will tell you that the act of sex came as a surprise, that they had not planned on having it happen. In fact, one recent study found that while they held values consistent with responsible sexual behavior, many teens did not translate those values into actual practice. Young people often lack the skills to resist peer pressures, to say NO to friends. It is not knowing how to assert their values that can lead some teens into trying and possibly abusing drugs or sex.

What?

Cigarettes • Alcohol • Marijuana • PCP • Cocaine
Heroin • LSD • Glue • Paint • Gasoline
Aerosol sprays • Chewing tobacco

Just about any substance you can name can be abused by adolescents. Certain drugs, however, are called "gateway drugs" because they do just that—provide a gateway to greater abuse. These gateway drugs include cigarettes, alcohol, and marijuana; all three are used by significant percentages of the young population. Some parents feel that they would actually be relieved to find that their child was "only smoking cigarettes" or using another less harmful substance. Unfortunately, their relief may be premature, for studies have shown that the youngster who abuses one substance is more likely to abuse a second or third substance as well. So if you happen to discover your child practicing one of these behaviors, check further to see if he or she is engaging in multiple substance abuse.

While teens living in different regions of the country practice different patterns of substance use, some trends are universal. In recent years, cigarette use has decreased among adolescent boys and increased among girls. Marijuana use has declined slightly. The most dramatic increase in drug use is seen for cocaine. The highest and most stable use, however, is seen for alcohol, which remains a significant problem.

Premarital sex and out-of-wedlock pregnancies have increased among teenagers. While premarital sex has been relatively common for young men, it has only recently become increasingly common for young women. Moreover, despite the greater sophistication and availability of contraceptives, teen pregnancies have reached epidemic proportions.

For many teens, the issue has become more complex than one of virginity or non-virginity. Rather, the issue is one of responsible sexual behavior and the ability to uphold personal values regarding sexual behavior. Intermixed with the issue of a healthy and appropriate sexuality is the renewed concern over sexually transmitted diseases. The risk of contracting gonorrhea, herpes, or AIDS is a hard fact that cannot be ignored.

When?

Is it true? Are our children growing up faster? If certain behaviors such as drug use or sex define growing up, then it may be so. Our children are trying drugs and sex at early ages.

The substances that children try first are generally cigarettes, alcohol, and marijuana. First use of these drugs typically begins during the preteen years and levels off by the midteen years. First use of "harder" drugs such as cocaine or psychedelics takes place at a somewhat later age, beginning during the midteen years and leveling off in early adulthood. Regular use of these substances tends to occur among older teens.

Among teens who have had intercourse, their first sexual act usually occurred during the midteens. On the average, girls report losing their virginity around age 16, and boys around age 15½. Black teens report having had their first intercourse at a younger age than white teens. The younger the teen, the less likely he or she used contraception during intercourse, thus increasing the likelihood of an unwanted pregnancy.

Where?

Geographically, drug use is generally highest among teens who live on either the East or West Coast. Some drugs are more popular in certain areas. For example, western teens use cocaine more frequently than teens in other areas of the country. Overall, urban teens appear to use more drugs than rural teens.

Within your own community there may be certain places that seem risky. Many parents worry too much about loud parties or the motel seduction scene. Certainly, these are among the places that teens may get involved in drugs or sex, but keep in mind that it is the teen and not the place that determines behavior. Moreover, loud parties are often no more that that—loud. And seedy motels are just as distasteful to teens as they are to adults.

Restricting a teen's mobility should not be a substitute for helping your teen develop values and the skills he needs to hold fast to those values. In fact, confining your son or daughter to a restricted location may be pointless when you consider that many young people find their home a convenient spot for improper behaviors. Teens can raid the home liquor cabinet, find a secluded room for smoking dope, or fit any unpermitted activity into the time they know the rest of the family will be away from home.

A likely spot to "get high" or " get laid" really depends on the individual community. Most young people know what parties, hang-outs, entertainment spots, and secluded areas should be off limits.

Putting the Pieces Together

Your teenager and his or her actions do not exist in isolation. Who your teen is and what he or she does fits into a much larger picture that includes the world around us as well as the world inside us. Therefore, any efforts to change or influence your teen must address the WHOLE picture: family relationships, other teens in the community, images we all get of the world through TV or other media, your child's natural development and curiosity, current or old problems your teen may be grappling with, and so on. As you read this book, you will begin to get a clearer picture of the world surrounding your child. But first, start thinking of your teen as an individual with individual feelings, individual dreams, individual stresses, and individual problems. Try a little empathy.

Who is that teenager living in your house? What has happened to the enjoyable child who seemed worlds away from thoughts of drugs or sex? Take heart, that enjoyable child still resides in your teenage son or daughter. What you see is a child trying to develop into an adult, at times succeeding and at times retreating.

Adolescence can be a time of vulnerable self-esteem when teens are unsure of themselves. In the early teen years, adolescents find esteem and security in practicing great conformity with their peers: they dress the same, talk the same, think the same. As the adolescent reaches the older teen years, he or she may try out roles to set him or herself apart from peers and from adults.

In any case, adolescents struggle toward the social and psychological goal of convincing the world that they are mature, confident, independent, and tough enough to make it on their own. A primary interest is to gain social skills, which they acquire from the world around them: peers, media, adults, and, of course, parents.

Adolescence is also a time of significant biological changes. To deny the existence of their sexual urges does not help adolescents cope with those urges in a healthy way. Moreover, consider for a moment how we are all bombarded by sexual messages in our culture. Our entertainment, advertisements, and the people around us often use sexual appeal to certain ends. The normal young person is tempted to respond to these influences. As a parent, you can help by instilling values and not just "laws", by finding outlets for teenage energies, by teaching skills for saying NO, and by providing warmth and affection.

The average teen will survive adolescence with relatively few problems. But even the average teen faces moments of temptation during periods of vulnerability. Like all of us, she stumbles through feelings of low self-esteem, confusion, and episodes of poor problem solving. She will naturally go through periods, generally brief, of being troubled. The truly troubled teen, however, has more difficulty bouncing back to firm grounding in identity, relationships with family and friends, and problem-solving capabilities.

Perhaps you can see how PREVENTING your teen from getting involved in sex or drugs can require a lot of cues and supports. Your teen's peers provide cues about acceptable behaviors. You too can be a cue in the type of role model you are, whether you drink or smoke too much, for example. You can provide support to your teen by teaching him how to think about consequences, by helping your teen be assertive in saying NO to pressures to behave in unacceptable ways, and by seeing your teen as a WHOLE person and not as a series of potential misbehaviors. And if your teen does stray, again consider the larger picture and not the isolated act. If you address only the act, then you may be putting a bandage on a wound that may not get better and may even get worse.

Let's look at a few examples. As you read these and other examples in the book, remember the old saying "Every story has two sides." Of course, we all realize that stories have far more than two sides; in the future, when you are about to respond to your teen's puzzling behavior, make it a habit to try thinking of not only two sides, but several. By having some insight into the reasons your child is doing something, you can better persuade him or her to change behaviors. Would having insight make a difference in how you would respond to the situation? It should. Of course, your immediate response might be anger or sadness. That's natural. You want your child to know that you disapprove and won't tolerate smoking, drinking, or sexual relations you deem inappropriate. Yet you also need to explore WHY he is practicing certain behaviors.

As you drive along the road one day, you see your son or daughter smoking cigarettes with friends. Before you throttle your teen, first ask why he or she might be smoking. The most common reason teens smoke is to fit in with friends, to be cool. This can be a healthy need, or it can stem from insecurity and poor relationships with peers that can lead your child to do something he or she doesn't really want to do. What if your child were smoking because:

1. He was curious about the taste and had never tried it.

7

2. She is addicted to cigarettes and has been smoking for two years.
3. He was trying to join a new group, and they all smoke.
4. She was mad at you for treating her like a child and, behind your back, wanted to "show you."
5. He felt worthless and unpopular and figured smoking might make him feel important.

Your 16-year-old comes home drunk from a dance. Again, some of the same reasons that cause the child above to smoke could lead him or her to drink. The problem may, however, extend more deeply and may certainly result in more serious immediate consequences, such as an accident.

1. What messages does she receive from you? What are your own drinking habits?
2. Does he fit a pattern of self-destructiveness that must be dealt with very seriously? Could he be an alcoholic?
3. Is he seeking an escape from any number of chronic problems such as failing in school or social circles?
4. Could she feel tense about dating and going to dances, which made her take a drink to relax?
5. Could he have wanted to celebrate a special occasion and got caught up in the spirit of the hour?

You are not certain, but you think your teenager is considering having sex, or may even have had sex. The young person who engages in sex at a young age may do so for a variety of reasons.

1. She feels unattractive or unloved.
2. He views sexual conquests as achievements to be proud of.
3. She is unable to say NO assertively, either because she is afraid or because she doesn't know how.
4. He doesn't know how to channel his sexual energies into alternative activities.
5. She has not made a mature decision about her sexual behavior based on well-considered attitudes and values.

How to Help

How can a parent help a child cope with decisions about drugs and sex? Where do you begin? Your concern is the best beginning. The very fact that you have picked up this book indicates concern and caring. By reading the rest of the book you can find out HOW to use your concern constructively and effectively. The short chapters and exercises are practical and down-to-earth.

We have two caveats before you begin: First, we all hold our own values about acceptable behaviors concerning drugs and sex. This book will not tell you what your values should be but it will help you define your values and share them with your family.

Second, you know your child better than we do. All youngsters differ—some struggle through adolescence, others sail through. Tailor the exercises and information to your own youngster's needs. Many children will enjoy the exercises in this book. Others might look at them with disdain. Encourage your child to try them. If your child is reluctant, you may need to be more spontaneous and creative in finding opportunities to get the point across. For example, you may need to point out situations that arise in the news, on TV, or among your child's friends, and ask what he would do in the situation or what he thinks about it.

This book is meant to give you action strategies, not just wisdom to think about certain behaviors. The exercises are designed to be used as an ongoing forum for practicing skills and for communicating. They are not meant to be "one-time-only" activities. Learn the skills presented in the exercises and use them often with your child. Your concern and willingness to learn is half the effort in helping to raise a healthy teen; your actions make up the other crucial half.

In the next chapter you will learn some techniques to help you communicate with your child. Talking to your child about drugs and sex helps him learn more about them from someone other than his peers. Try to be informed about these topics or at least know where to get accurate information. Having knowledge about drugs and sex is not detrimental to your child; it is the lack of knowledge that can be harmful.

KIDS, DRUGS, AND SEX

You can never start too early in establishing open communications with your child. Do not wait until your child asks about these important issues. Some children never do, others may not know how.

2

HOW TO TALK TO YOUR CHILD

The eyes are glazed and fixed on a distant target. The shoulders are hunched. The face remains motionless except for an occasional blink of the eye or sniffing of the nose. There is little sign of bodily movement—just a brief scratching at the neck or arm. Hardly any indication of life. No response to verbal stimuli except a disconcerting "Huh? What did you say?"

Diagnosis: "Catatonic Incommunicado." Commonly known in lay terms as selective listening, parentally induced deafness, or the "hasn't heard a single word" syndrome.

Prognosis: Very good with proper attention to developing good communication skills. (Note: The disorder may eventually disappear once the patient has children of his or her own, but parents are advised not to wait that long.)

There is really no disorder called "Catatonic Incommunicado," but, according to many parents, there *should* be such a term. If your child suffers from the above malady, it is time to seek a cure. Even if your child does not manifest these symptoms, there may be other less evident ones. Let's face it, almost all families could stand to improve their communication skills. Do you really know the people who live in the house with you? Do you really listen to them? Do they listen to you? How do they feel about important issues? Can you even discuss those issues?

The issues raised in this book—drugs and sex—are not always

easy to discuss. You must first make sure you know how to talk to your child before you can comfortably discuss these topics or help him learn the skills he will need to deal with them. The ability to communicate is the foundation of any solid relationship and it must be laid with care. This chapter describes the basic components of good communication skills and provides suggestions on how you and your child can improve your skills.

The Process

What happens when you talk to your child? At a minimum, communication requires three main components: a sender (parent), a receiver (child), and a message. The sender transmits a message, which is picked up by the receiver.

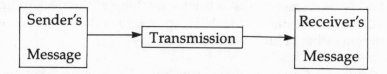

This looks pretty simple. Unfortunately, many interferences can occur during transmission and lead to MISUNDERSTAND-INGS. We have all experienced the frustration of being misunderstood. Misunderstandings can be caused by the sender or by the receiver; they can quickly disrupt communication. Let's take a look at how misunderstandings might happen in a hypothetical situation.

It is getting dark outside, dinner is on the table, and Roger is not home from school yet. Mother is worried about him. He did not mention anything about coming home late. Roger bounds in the door yelling, "What's for dinner?" Mother is both relieved and angry, and she wants to know where he has been. She also wants Roger to tell her ahead of time when he is going to be late.

There are several ways that Roger or Mother might react to this situation that could lead to a misunderstanding:

Source of Misunderstanding	*Example*
The message is stated too vaguely.	Mother says "Your dinner is cold!" instead of asking why Roger was late.
The receiver is formulating his own argument instead of listening.	Roger is thinking of excuses and does not hear that his mother is concerned about his safety.
The nonverbal message conflicts with the verbal one.	Mother greets Roger with a frozen smile and says,"I'm glad you're home."
The message falls on deaf ears.	Roger bolts upstairs to his room just as Mother begins to talk.

In the examples above, both Roger and his mother were responsible for the misunderstandings that arose, because they did not make the *effort* to understand. Maybe they could have clarified things immediately by taking a moment to talk:

Mother: Roger, I was so worried about you. Where were you?
Roger: I was at Tim's house and didn't realize the time. I tried to call but the line was busy, so I ran home.
Mother: Please let me know if you're going to be late in the future, and tell me where you plan to be so I can call if you're not home on time.
Roger: I will, Mom. Next time I'll call first to let you know where I am.

That seems simple. Mother talks to Roger, Roger responds to Mother, and they both understand each other. It is *too* simple. Communication is rarely as simple as one person telling something to another. Communication is a complex system of influences and inferences. To the simple picture of sender, transmission, and receiver, we must add the weight of any problems or fears that bother the sender or receiver, such as preconceptions and memories of past communications or events.

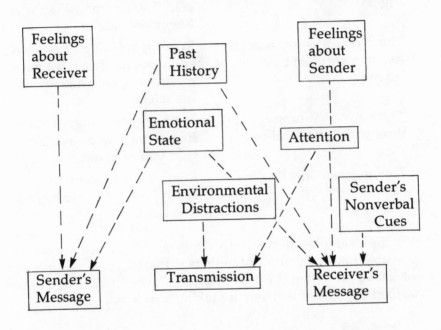

In the example of Roger and his mother, we can add these possible scenarios:

- Roger has been late three times this week and keeps promising to call beforehand to tell his mother where he will be.
- Mother always refuses permission to stay out when Roger does ask her.
- Tim has been caught smoking marijuana and Roger has been forbidden to go to his house.
- A child was kidnapped as he was walking home from school in a neighboring community last week.

The outside world may add to the complexity and confusion. Other people may be present, either obstructing your message or adding to it. The communication between Roger and his mother might have been different if:

- the phone had started ringing
- Father had intervened with "Let's not argue. Dinner is ready."
- a pot on the stove had started boiling over
- Roger had turned up the stereo

As the diagram on page 14 suggests, the "simple act" of communicating can become very complex. That is why it takes a strong commitment to really make it work.

It seems that once misunderstandings start, they tend to snowball into larger arguments. Neither side feels understood and both sides feel pretty hopeless about the potential for being understood. In these kinds of standoffs, people usually react by either attacking or retreating.

Attacking consists of blaming the other side for the lack of communication. ("You never listen to me." "You never talk to me.") Retreating is characterized primarily by silence, accompanied by reluctance or dread of being in the same room with the other side. ("What's the use, we don't have anything in common." "Let's just drop it, okay?")

Needless to say, both the reactions of attacking and retreating are just that, *reactions*. To break the unproductive circle, you must *act*, not surrender to your reactions.

What Can I Do?

There are four basic steps to improving your chances of having a meaningful conversation with your child.

C—COMMUNICATE
A—ATTEND
R—REFLECT
E—ENCOURAGE

As the acronym suggests, you have to CARE enough to take the initiative. Communication is a two-way street, though the desire to communicate may be very one-sided at first. This is understandable, particularly if past efforts have been less than successful. Do not give up. By examining and improving your own skills

15

at communicating, you provide a more comfortable environment in which your child can feel safer and more relaxed about communicating. Essentially, your goal is to become "someone who's easy to talk to."

By taking the initiative to improve your own ability to communicate, you actively demonstrate a commitment. You are saying to your child, "Being able to understand you is so important to me that I am willing to examine my own behavior and make changes." When you actively practice good communication skills, you become a role model for your child. He may in time, with guidance and encouragement, become adept at using these skills himself! But first things first. Let's examine each of the four steps to good communication.

C-Communicate

COMMUNICATE YOUR MESSAGES
CLEARLY AND HONESTLY

This section deals with your role as sender. The message you send should be a simple, direct statement of the thoughts or feelings you want to convey. This is easier said than done, for it requires that you be fully aware of your thoughts and feelings. Here are some rules on how to be a good sender:

1. Keep it simple. Talk about one topic at a time.
2. Focus on the here and now. Try to avoid dredging up past issues—they only detract from the topic at hand.
3. Think before you speak. Formulate exactly what you want to say before you say it.
4. Consider ways you might be misinterpreted and try to express yourself in ways that avoid misinterpretations.
5. Put yourself in the receiver's shoes. How would you react to the message? Is there a better way to say it?
6. Make sure your nonverbal message says the same thing that your words say.
7. Face the receiver and maintain good eye contact. Don't stare at the person, just look at him frequently.
8. Express how you are feeling.

Consider the following situation:

Kevin had just received his report card with a very low grade in math. He felt ashamed and scared, and he left the card on his father's desk to be signed. When Father saw it, he was angry and disappointed, but he hid these feelings by acting very logically and rationally. In a matter-of-fact way, he went into Kevin's room and announced, "I want to talk to you about your school work and about how you're doing with your chores at home. Last week you didn't mow the lawn and the week before you were two hours late getting home from school. Your grade in math was lousy. It looks like you've got a lot of shaping up to do."

Look at the list above. Which rules did father violate?

Rule 1: He had a list of topics a mile long, not just the report card.
Rule 2: The list stretched back two weeks.
Rule 5: Father didn't stop to consider how Kevin must be feeling about the grade, or how much worse he would feel by hearing about all his other mistakes.
Rule 8: Instead of expressing his own feelings, Father put up a very formal facade, which made it pretty difficult for Kevin to open up.

What could Father have done instead? First, he needs to decide what message he really wants to send and focus on that. Second, he needs to express his own feelings. Third, he needs to consider how Kevin might be feeling and decide on the best way to get his message across to Kevin. A more direct way of handling the situation might have been to say:

"Kevin, I just saw your grade in math and I'm angry and disappointed. I imagine you're feeling pretty bad too. I'd like to talk to you about why you got such a low grade and what you can

17

do to improve next semester. I know you're capable of doing better and if you need some help from me, you've got it. But first, tell me what you think about it."

Father was very clear about his disappointment, but he left the door open for Kevin to talk too. The message was clear, honest, and CARING.

Exercise 1 is designed to help you analyze communications. Acquaint yourself with the rules for being a good communicator and become aware of times when those rules are ignored. Think of more effective ways to get your message across.

A-Attend

PAY CLOSE ATTENTION TO WHAT IS BEING SAID

Now the other side of the conversation, your role as receiver. This section focuses more on developing good listening skills than on communicating your own messages effectively. This is because your ability to be a good listener will make it easier for your child to share his thoughts and feelings with you. The goal is to develop good communications with your child; the best way to do this is to become the kind of person your child *wants* to talk to.

The role of listener is definitely the most difficult for some parents. To learn it well you must keep a careful watch on your listening or "attending" skills. The good listener:

- truly desires to understand others
- gives the speaker her undivided attention
- never interrupts the speaker
- faces the speaker and maintains good eye contact
- gives an occasional nod or "uh huh" to reassure the speaker that he understands
- absorbs both the content and the feeling of what is said

Think about those characteristics as you read the scenario that follows on page 20.

Exercise 1   **PARENT**

ANALYZING COMMUNICATIONS

Reread the list of eight rules for good communications on page 16. Then read the following scenario, decide which rules were broken, and think of a better way to communicate the message.

Heather's mother called her into the kitchen to talk to her. Mother was washing the dishes and facing out the window as she spoke:

"Heather, your sister told me you wore her sweater today without her permission. You are never to do that again, do you understand? That was inconsiderate. You've been doing a lot of inconsiderate things lately. You forgot to clean up your mess in the kitchen and I had to do it, and you monopolize the phone all the time so no one else can use it."

Which rules did Mother break? Give examples. (Answers below.)

_____

_____

_____

_____

_____

_____

_____

What could Mother have said to communicate her message more clearly? _____

_____

_____

_____

_____

Answers: The following rules were broken:

Rule 1—Mother talked about several topics (sweater, mess, phone).
Rule 2—She brought up grievances from the past.
Rule 4—It is unclear whether Heather should never wear the sweater or whether she can only do so if she gets permission.
Rule 5—Mother was pretty insensitive to Heather's feelings.
Rule 7—She did not face Heather while speaking.
Rule 8—Mother did not express her feelings.

Mary had a habit of looking away whenever her son spoke to her. She would continue doing her needlepoint or working in the kitchen, very rarely making eye contact with her son. She realized that in their conversations her son would often ask whether she had heard him and she frequently repeated, "Yes, I'm still listening." Mary's son initiated fewer and fewer conversations with her, and the ones he did start became shorter and shorter.

The problem really hit home for Mary one day when she went to her son's room to talk to him while he was watching television. She talked while her son, nodding occasionally, stared at the TV. Mary felt herself getting more and more irritated and finally burst out with, "Look at me when I'm talking to you!" She was unprepared for her son's equally vehement response, "Why should I? *You* never do!"

Mary began to look at her own behavior and realized that her son was right. She was often preoccupied with other things when someone else was talking. Even though she reassured others that she was still listening, she noticed that people spent less time talking to her when they didn't have her full attention. When she asked her husband to give her feedback, he admitted that she often looked away while he was talking to her and that he felt unimportant or boring when she did that. Mary decided to pay closer ATTENTION to people by practicing better listening skills.

R-Reflect

REFLECT BACK WHAT YOU HAVE JUST HEARD

Perhaps the most important part of communicating is to "reflect back" what you have just heard. It is the only way to be sure that the receiver truly undersands what the sender is saying. When you reflect back what is being said, you give the sender your interpretation of the message to make sure it is the same as his.

Child: I really hate spending every Saturday visiting Grandma.
Parent: You hate it? What is it you hate?
Child: It's boring.

Exercise 2   **PARENT**

LISTENING SKILLS INVENTORY

Becoming a good listener requires an objective understanding of your strengths and weaknesses.

Directions: After your next conversation with your child, ask yourself the following questions. Write "yes" or "no" next to each number to indicate your answer.

1. Did you interrupt at any time?
2. Did you talk longer than your child?
3. Did you look at him (her) when he (she) spoke?
4. Did you become distracted during the conversation?
5. If you had to guess what your child was feeling, would you have had a good idea?
6. While your child was speaking, were your thoughts ever centered on what you would say in response?
7. Did you try to finish your child's sentences for her (him)?
8. Did you nod or show some sign of understanding?
9. Was understanding your child the most important thing on your mind at that moment?
10. Were you calm and relaxed while listening?
11. Could you accurately restate what you just heard?

If you answered "Yes" to questions 1, 2, 4, 6, or 7, put a circle around those numbers that got a "Yes."

If you answered "No" to questions 3, 5, 8, 9, 10, or 11, put a circle around those numbers that got a "No."

Go back and look at the numbers you circled. These are the areas where you might need some improvement. (Be sure to look at the items that were not circled to see where your strengths lie.)

When you feel you are ready for some feedback about your listening skills, ask your child (or whomever was speaking to you) to rate your behavior as a listener.

21

Parent: You think Grandma is boring?
Child: Not Grandma. It's just that there's nothing to do and I can't be with my friends.
Parent: You don't think Grandma is boring. It's just that you miss spending time with your friends and there's nothing that interests you at her house.
Child: Yeah. I miss listening to my music and practicing basketball.
Parent: What if we brought your radio along? We could even bring the basketball and drive over to the schoolyard after lunch and shoot baskets for a while.
Child: That would be a lot better.
Parent: And maybe we could arrange to let you stay with your friends one Saturday when there's some special activity going on.
Child: Great!

By reflecting back what has just been said, you (a) show the sender that you are really paying attention, (b) avoid jumping to the wrong conclusions, and (c) are better able to respond to the message that was sent. This process is particularly helpful in dealing with conflicts, because it forces each person to "see the other's side" before presenting another view.

The ability to accurately reflect is an art that requires much practice. Many people feel reluctant to try it because they think it will sound artificial or contrived. "If I parrot back what I just heard, she'll think I'm getting senile." "It sounds so strange." "I heard what he said. Why do I have to repeat it?"

Try it anyway. You will find that once you get comfortable with it, your reflections will sound natural. Others will probably feel flattered that you CARE enough to understand them and they will often make more of an effort to return the favor.

Steps for Reflecting Back

Step 1: Take a moment to let the message sink in.
Step 2: Think of another way of saying what you have just heard, or "paraphrase" the message.

Step 3: Present your interpretation of the message back to the sender.

Step 4: Make sure the paraphrased message is the same as what the sender intended to say.

Step 5: Deliver your own message in response to what you heard.

Here are two examples of communications between a parent and child, one that involves misunderstandings and one that uses reflection to avoid misunderstandings.

Example 1—Misunderstandings

Son: Dad, the guys invited me to go to a football game this Saturday. I know you wanted me to mow the lawn on Saturday, but we would have to leave really early to get to the game and we wouldn't be home till dark.

Father: I suppose you expect me to do your work for you while you go off and have a good time. Forget it!

Son: Wait, Dad, you're not being fair. I plan to . . . .

Father: You heard what I said. You can't go! I've got other things to do besides taking care of your chores.

In this example, the father jumped to the conclusion that his son wanted him to mow the lawn. The son felt that he had been misunderstood and treated unfairly. Both parties left the conversation feeling angry.

Example 2—Trying to Understand

Son: Dad, the guys invited me to go to a football game this Saturday. I know you wanted me to mow the lawn on Saturday, but we would have to leave really early to get to the game and we wouldn't be home till dark.

Father: It sounds like you want to go to the game, but it conflicts with your chores.

Son: Yes, that's right. Can I mow the lawn later?

Father: You want to mow the lawn later? How much later?
Son: How about if I go to the game and mow the lawn the next day?
Father: Your solution is to delay mowing the lawn for one day? That sounds okay with me.

In this example, the father accurately reflected back the son's dilemma and asked him to come up with a solution. He paraphrased the solution, to "mow the lawn later," and asked his son to clarify what he meant by "later". This forced the son to devise a more specific solution that they could both accept. Both parties felt that they had been understood and that they had reached an agreement.

By reflecting back what you have heard, you get a chance to check the accuracy of your perceptions about what has been said. Sometimes we can be too quick in making assumptions about what the sender is saying. This invariably leads to misunderstandings and interferes with good communications. Reflecting is one way of trying to prevent these misunderstandings.

E-Encourage

PROVIDE ENCOURAGEMENT AND PRAISE

When was the last time you complimented your child on something he did well? When was the last time you criticized him for something he did wrong? People are often a lot better at criticizing than complimenting. This is unfortunate because compliments and encouragement not only tell a child what he is doing that is right, they also help to build a positive self-esteem.

A child's sense of self-esteem is often closely linked with his parents' evaluations and expectations of him. When children are complimented and encouraged, they begin to feel good about themselves, trusting their own abilities and developing confidence in themselves. They are more open and relaxed in communicating with others and feel good about those who encourage them.

24

By contrast, children who are criticized and discouraged from trying new things feel unsure of themselves. They tend to be more timid and quiet. They also try to protect themselves from experiencing failure, either by avoiding challenges or by closing themselves off from those who criticize them.

When communicating with your child, consider your child's self-esteem. Obviously you would not want to tell her that everything she does is wonderful, just as you would not tell her that everything she does is terrible. Criticisms and compliments are part of learning to deal with the world and parents must use both with their children. Here are a few pointers to use when communicating with your child that may help to enhance his or her self-esteem.

1. Be sure to catch your child doing the right thing and let her know it. Too often we focus on the negative and fail to reward the positive behaviors.
2. If you must criticize, make it brief and specific. Say exactly what was wrong about a behavior and let your child know what an acceptable, alternative behavior might be.
3. Be sure to criticize the behavior and not the person. Always let your child know that even though you disapprove of the bad behavior, you still love him.
4. Compliment your child about things that are important to her. Find out your child's goals and dreams and encourage her attempts to fulfill them.
5. Make your compliments meaningful. Look your child in the eye and touch him when you give him a compliment.
6. Always finish a criticism with an encouragement. Tell your child you know she will do the right thing next time.
7. Try to give your child more compliments than criticisms. Make sure your statements are balanced more toward the positive than the negative of your child's self-esteem. ,

Parents can greatly influence their child's self-esteem, depending upon whether they *encourage* or *discourage* their child. Self-esteem, belief in one's own abilities, confidence, personal aspirations—these are all part of a child's identity and all are easily affected by parents. Consider the examples below:

Example 1

Susie brought home an excellent report card and showed it to her mother.

Encouraging Mother: Susie, that's wonderful! I'm so proud of you. Wait until your father sees this report card.

Discouraging Mother: Yes, dear, that's very good. But then I wouldn't expect anything but good grades. Now if you could only do as well at keeping your room clean.

Example 2

Janet brought home a mediocre report card, with two bad grades and two good grades, and showed it to her father.

Encouraging Father: I'm concerned about your grades in science and English. I know you can do better than that with a little extra work. Those are good grades you got in math and history. I'm proud of you for the work you did to get them.

Discouraging Father: Those are lousy grades you got. You're just being lazy and not studying enough. You can't watch any TV until you bring home a good report card and prove to me you're not stupid.

Which reaction, encouraging or discouraging, will most likely make Susie and Janet enthusiastic about school and about getting good grades?

Parents who encourage their children develop stronger and more trusting relationships with them. Children communicate more openly in a nurturing environment because they feel that their parents are more their allies than their adversaries.

Start to Communicate—Start to CARE

Becoming a better communicator requires the same patience and practice that goes with learning any new skill. To begin, review the list of communication skills under each of the CARE sections.

Ask yourself which you do well and which you do poorly or not at all. Ask someone you trust to give you feedback about your skills. Does he or she have suggestions about areas for improvement? Ask your child to give you feedback too. After all, it is important to know how your child perceives your ability to communicate. It also lets your child know that you CARE about him and want to know more about him.

Take Time. Learning to communicate, getting to know each other, building a stronger relationship—these all take time. Be more available to your child and initiate conversations more often. Be sensitive to her desires and don't force a conversation.

Set aside a specific time, on a regular basis, to talk with your child and practice being a good listener. Sometimes it helps to set an "appointment" with your child and hold your conversation in a comfortable location. Make sure you set a time and a place that are agreeable to both you and your child.

Some Tips on What to Say

Ask questions about the things that interest your child. The best kinds of questions are "open-ended"—those that require a full statement rather than a mere "yes" or "no" response.

Open-ended question: What do you think about the teachers you have this year in school?
Close-ended question: Do you like the teachers you have this year in school?

Open-ended question: If you could do anything you wanted for a career, what jobs would appeal to you?
Close-ended question: Do you think you'd like to become a lawyer like your mother?

Choose A Skill To Work On. After you have reviewed the CARE lists and identified specific skills you would like to improve or develop, choose just one that you want to work on first. It is best to choose a fairly simple skill to begin with.

For example, by conducting a self-assessment, you may have

found yourself less than perfect in your ATTENDING skills. Don't vow to become the perfect listener in one day. Instead, set a smaller, more specific goal, such as increasing eye contact. Think about making eye contact in every conversation you have with your child, your spouse, your boss, the cashier, the bank teller. Get started with one skill, and you will notice that other skills will follow.

Regularly Reassess. How are you doing? Are your skills improving? Maybe you've mastered eye contact and you're ready to tackle more or more complex skills. Or maybe you're not doing that well and need to go back to basics and choose simpler skills.

You must constantly reassess your skills. One easy way to do this is to review the lists of CARE skills periodically and see how they compare with your own behavior in a recent conversation. Another way is to ask other people, particularly your child, to tell you how you're doing. This may be uncomfortable or awkward, but when you open up to someone and ask for their opinions about you, you're often setting the stage for close and meaningful communications.

Now Is The Time. There is no better time than right now. If you put it off or hope something will intervene to improve your ability to communicate, you are deluding yourself. You can't afford to wait until your child grows up; there is too much at stake in the growing period. Go ahead, give it a try.

What if it Still Doesn't Work?

So you've tried repeatedly to open the channels of communication with your child, but you just can't seem to reach her. Now what? First, keep a cool head. Parent-child relationships can be difficult at times but that doesn't mean the difficulties are insurmountable.

Look In Your Own Backyard First. What you must avoid is placing the blame on that kid of yours. We too often make the mistake that "it's the other person's fault." It is hard to look critically at ourselves, but it is easier to change ourselves than to change others. Many people in troubled relationships learn that the only true control an individual has is over self, not over the other person or over the dynamics of the relationship.

Ask yourself how honest you are being with your child.

- Are you using the techniques in this chapter to really get to know your child, or are you using them to manipulate her?
- Are you really listening to your child? Do you understand what he is telling you, either in words or silence?
- Are you trying hard enough to put yourself in your child's place? Empathy is the highway to communication.
- Are you expecting miracles? Patience is more than a virtue; it's usually a key to real success. Don't expect open communication channels after only a few tries, and don't expect open channels to stay open if you don't persist. Remember to be persistent, but not insistent.

Changing the Relationship. If you can honestly say you've tried your best yet still can't reach your child, or if you feel too many obstacles prevent you from doing your best, then you may have to rely on people outside yourself and your child, particularly if you are worried or have reason to believe your child might be in trouble. Here are some suggestions:

1. Find a third party both you and your child respect and trust. The third party might be the other parent or an older sibling who may have a better relationship with the child. A close relative or neighbor can help as well. This person can act as interpreter for both you and your child. The eventual goal is for the third party to help the two of you become closer. But be careful what you ask of the other person: being in the middle can be a touchy spot—you are asking a lot of someone.
2. Ask an objective outsider to intervene. A school counselor, pastor, coach, or other authoritative adult can provide more formal repair of your communication channels.

3. Seek professional counseling. Never overlook the help of a trained therapist. If you have any personal fears about psychological counseling or consider it a last resort in only hopeless situations, cast such feelings away. You are dealing with too important an issue to let personal prejudice and misinformation stand in the way.

Communicating about Drugs and Sex

In many ways, your communication skills will affect how well you and your child are able to talk about the issues of drugs and sexuality. As the two of you complete the exercises presented in the following chapters, use these opportunities to work on your communication skills. Try to become a parent who is easy to approach and easy to talk to.

3

IT'S HOW YOU SAY IT

Your ability to communicate with other people varies from day to day. Some days you may be eloquent, with words tripping off your tongue; on other days it seems that no matter what you say, it comes out the wrong way. Some days you may be softspoken, withdrawn, or tense; other days you may be loud, gregarious, or cheerful.

While everyone experiences these variations, most people tend to demonstrate a consistent "style" of communicating. Communication styles are often learned early in life. Many people feel that they can never change, others are fearful of trying new styles, still others fiercely defend their style as the best without examining the alternatives.

The truth of the matter is that sometimes it's not what you say, it's how you say it. We can identify four major communication styles. Everyone has used each style at one time or another; nonetheless, each of us tends to use one style more often. Before we examine the four communication styles, read the statements below and see if they remind you of people you know.

1. Tom is too pushy. He always has to have his own way.
2. I never know what Mary really wants. She always gives in to avoid a disagreement.
3. Jack says one thing but does another. He gives in to others, but tries to make them feel guilty about it the whole time.
4. Liz gives her opinion openly, but always seems to care about mine too.

31

Do you know people who fit any of these descriptions? Which describes you the best? We all use different styles of communicating at different times, but, for the most part, people fall into one of four categories: Aggressive, Passive, Assertive, or Passive-Aggressive. Each style has its own verbal and nonverbal characteristics.

What happens when people use each of the response styles? Do they get what they want? How do other people feel? How do they feel about themselves? What do other people think about them?

The Aggressive Person

This person often gets his own way, but at great expense. He makes lots of demands and seldom thinks about anyone else's thoughts or feelings. People often avoid him and consider him overbearing and a bully. He makes people feel angry or hurt and sometimes feels guilty about it later. This person seems to care only about himself, which doesn't leave much room for others to care about him.

Verbal Responses
Makes demands; doesn't listen to others or take their feelings into account; sometimes insulting or angry; self-centered speech

Nonverbal Responses
Loud voice; stares or glares; doesn't let others talk very much; rigid posture, tense muscles; looks angry or hurried

The Passive Person

This person will do almost anything to avoid an argument. She is so afraid of hurting other people that she bends over backwards to agree with them. Often this means that her own needs do not get met. People tend to take advantage of her and think of her as a "pushover" or a "jellyfish." They often get frustrated because they never know what she really wants. She often feels frustrated herself because she doesn't express her opinions or desires and later wishes she had. Her self-esteem is often low. People don't take her needs seriously because she doesn't.

Verbal Responses
Often gives in or backs down when pressured; doesn't express feelings and opinions openly; qualifies statements with "maybe" or "I think"

Nonverbal Responses
Doesn't maintain eye contact; often looks down; doesn't stand up straight; soft voice; looks nervous or timid

The Passive-Aggressive Person

This person appears cooperative and gracious on the surface, deferring to others and giving in to their requests. In many ways, he is like the passive person who fails to express his own needs. But there is one important difference—although he gives in at the time, he later gets back at other people in subtle or indirect ways. If he doesn't want to do something, he will agree to do it when you ask but fail to carry through with it. This person probably creates the most anger and frustration among others because no one really knows what to expect. Others distrust him and do not respect him. He often feels smug and self-satisfied when he refuses to follow through with his promises. He justifies his behavior by blaming the other person for "having the nerve to ask that of me."

Verbal Responses
Gives in at the moment; later attacks or blames others and fails to keep commitments

Nonverbal Responses
Similar to the passive style; sometimes has a "cold" expression or phony smile

The Assertive Person

This person speaks her mind but she does so in such a way that she doesn't criticize or take advantage of other people. She views disagreement not as a disaster but as a challenge—"Can we come up with a solution that we can both accept?" She is straightforward, honest, and, at the same time, considerate of how others feel. Others respect her. They never have to "second guess" what she is trying to say, because they know she will tell them her true thoughts and feelings. She feels confident and good about herself.

Verbal Responses
Expresses thoughts and feelings openly; solicits others' opinions; listens to others; not hesitant to stand up for own rights but protects others' rights too

Nonverbal Responses
Speaks clearly and confidently; calm and relaxed posture; stands up straight; pleasant facial expression and good eye contact

Looking at each of the styles, it is pretty clear that the ASSERTIVE person seems to be the most effective in communicating her thoughts and the most successful in gaining the respect of others. Learning to be assertive is often difficult, because it goes against some of the things people are taught. We learn many poor communication styles, which makes it that much harder to relearn better ones.

Girls are often told to be sweet and kind, and never to "make a fuss" (PASSIVE). Boys may be told to fight for themselves, to go after what they want, "may the best man win" (AGGRESSIVE). Children are frequently told to obey and not question their elders, so they sometimes agree to do something and "conveniently forget" (PASSIVE-AGGRESSIVE).

Teaching your child to be more assertive means that you cannot have "total control" over the situation. Assertiveness means that your child must think for himself and express his own ideas, even if they conflict with yours. This does not mean that your child should always get his way, but it does mean that he should be encouraged to express differences of opinion.

Some parents do not want their children to express their thoughts and feelings. They would prefer that their children simply follow orders and never question what they say. While this may be easier for the parent, it tends to create low self-esteem and little confidence among children.

Exercise 3   **PARENT and CHILD**

RECOGNIZING THE STYLES

Below are some examples of the different communication styles. Each one represents a different response to the same request. In the space at the left of each statement, put the number of the style it represents.

1 = Aggressive
2 = Passive
3 = Passive-Aggressive
4 = Assertive

Your friend asked if s/he could borrow your new sweater to wear to a big party on Saturday. You just bought the sweater and don't want to lend it to your friend. You say:

__(A) "Well, I guess it would be okay."

__(B) "Borrow my new sweater? Are you crazy? You'd probably destroy it before I even get a chance to wear it."

__(C) "Sure you can wear it. I bet it will look great on you." When Saturday comes around you say, "Oh, I'm sorry. I forgot to pick it up from the cleaner's and they're closed now."

__(D) "I'd rather not lend you my new sweater. I haven't worn it myself yet."

__(E) "You've got some nerve. Why don't you go out and buy your own sweater?"

__(F) "Oh that sweater? I'd be glad to lend it to you but it isn't mine. I borrowed it from someone else."

__(G) "I guess you can wear it. Do you want to wear the new shoes I bought to go with it?"

__(H) "I know you want to look special on Saturday, but I just bought that sweater and I want to be the first to wear it. Let's see if I've got something else you'd like to wear."

__(I) "Sure. You'll look great in it." Later to another friend: "S/he practically grabbed it out of my hands. What a jerk!"

Answers: A-2; B-1; C-3; D-4; E-1; F-3; G-2; H-4; I-3

The child who is taught to obey without questioning never learns how to make independent, mature decisions. He never learns how to decide what is good or bad for him, because someone else has always done that. When he leaves home, he may still let others make his decisions or influence what he does. Unlike his parents, they may not have his best interests at heart.

If a child is taught to obey blindly, how do you think he might respond to pressures to take drugs or engage in sex? Certainly not by standing up for what he truly believes—he has never learned how to stand up for what he believes nor to decide what he truly believes!

How can you help your child become more assertive? First, you can both become more aware of the different communication styles. Second, you can analyze your own communication styles and decide how you might like to change them. Third, you can practice being more assertive with each other. And fourth, you can catch each other being assertive and give praise and encouragement.

Exercises 4, 5, and 6 are for you to complete with your child. They will help the two of you learn to be more assertive. Exercise 4 presents situations that might occur in everyday life and asks you both to give examples of the different response styles so that you will become familiar with them. Exercise 5 presents situations with drug- or sex-related themes and asks you and your child to give assertive responses. Exercise 6 gives suggestions on how you can continue to use your new skills daily.

A Final Word to Parents

At the same time you encourage your child to be assertive, be so yourself. Parents sometimes find it difficult to find the right way of communicating. They may be either too aggressive or too passive.

Be honest with your feelings and attitudes. If you are angry with, or hurt by, your child, say so. If you think she is doing something wrong, say so. On the other hand, be honest with positive feelings as well. Don't try to hide your feelings and beliefs behind a wall of "communication techniques."

Exercise 4   **PARENT and CHILD**

WHAT CAN I SAY?

There are many different styles of communicating. Review the description of the four styles presented in this chapter: Aggressive, Passive, Passive-Aggressive, and Assertive.

In each of the situations below, think of a response that would fit each style. An example is provided at the beginning. After you have read the example, read the other situations aloud and take turns thinking of different styles of responding to the situations. Write your answers next to they styles they represent.

Example

SITUATION: You have just eaten dinner at a nice restaurant and the waitress brings you the check. She has added the bill incorrectly and has overcharged you by about five dollars.

POSSIBLE RESPONSES
Aggressive: (to the waitress) "What are you trying to do, rip me off? I'm not going to pay for your mistakes!"
Passive: (to yourself) "I don't want to make a fuss. I'll just pay it. The dinner was worth more anyway."
Passive-Aggressive: (to yourself) "I'll pay the bill and not say anything, but I certainly won't leave her any tip! I'll never come here again!"
Assertive: (to the waitress) "There seems to be a mistake on this check. Will you please add it again?"

Your Turn

Now you try it. Remember, the way you say it often determines what the response style is, so when you answer, make sure your tone fits the style.

(continued)

(*Exercise 4 continued*)

SITUATION: A telephone salesman calls you and pressures you to buy a magazine subscription. You have no interest in the magazine, and you think it is much too expensive.

POSSIBLE RESPONSES
Aggressive: (to   ) _____

_____

Passive: (to   ) _____

_____

Passive-Aggressive: (to   ) _____

_____

Assertive: (to   ) _____

_____

SITUATION: You are riding the elevator to the top floor of an office building. Someone gets on at the second floor smoking a cigarette. The smoke really bothers you and you know it's against the law to smoke in an elevator.

POSSIBLE RESPONSES
Aggressive: (to   ) _____

_____

Passive: (to   ) _____

_____

Passive-Aggressive: (to   ) _____

_____

Assertive: (to   ) _____

_____

Now read the following questions and discuss your answers:

1. In each of the situations above, which communication style would probably work best?
2. How do you think others would react to the different responses you wrote? (Go back and review the responses.)
3. Which style do you honestly think you would use in each of the situations above?

Exercise 5   **PARENT and CHILD**

BEING ASSERTIVE

The following is a structured exercise designed to increase awareness about social pressures and provide practice in standing up for your rights. Parents should read the first two situations to their children and ask the questions following each situation. (Note: Different situations are provided for preteens and teenagers.) Be sure to record the answers given.

Next, the tables are turned and children must read the third and fourth situations to their parents. Ask the questions that follow and record the answers. Finally, both parents and their children should answer the questions at the end of the exercise together.

Preteens

SITUATION 1 (Parent reads to child)
"After school, you and several classmates go over to a friend's house to play. Your friend's mother leaves to go to the grocery store and your friend says, 'While she's gone, let's sneak one of her cigarettes and smoke it in the bathroom. She'll never know.' You feel uncomfortable and don't want to smoke."

How could you be assertive in expressing your thoughts and feelings in this situation?_____

Would you stay or would you leave? _____
Why? _____
What could I do in this situation to make things easier for you?

_____

(continued)

(*Exercise 5 continued*)

SITUATION 2 (Parent reads to child)
"Pretend that a friend of yours has just found a 'dirty' magazine, full of naked people. Your friend is afraid that his/her parents might find the magazine and asks if you will hide it in your bedroom for a few days. You don't want to do it, but your friend keeps begging."

How could you express your thoughts and feelings assertively? _____

What do you think you would do in this situation? _____
_____

How do you think I might react if I found the magazine? _____

Teenagers

SITUATION 1 (Parent reads to child)
"Pretend that you have been invited to a party at a friend's house. When you get there, you find that your friend's parents have gone out of town. Other people have brought lots of beer and marijuana to the party and they are trying to get you to join them in drinking and smoking."

How could you express your thoughts and feelings in an assertive way? _____

Would you stay or would you leave? _____

Why? _____

What could I do to help you in this situation? _____
_____

SITUATION 2 (Parent reads to child. Intended for child of either sex)
"You have just gone out on a date with someone you've just met. You really like this person a lot and want to go out with him/her again. You are in the car talking before going home, and your date starts to make advances and suggests you two get more intimate than you want to."

(*continued*)

(*Exercise 5 continued*)

What would you do? _____

What if this person refused to go out with you again unless
you went along with his/her demands? _____

_____

What if this person teased you or called you a baby?

_____

What could you do if that person became aggressive or tried
to force you to do something you didn't want to do?

_____

How could you avoid this situation in the future?_____

_____

Parents

SITUATION 3 (Child reads to parents)
"Imagine you have gone out to dinner with some friends.
You had some drinks at dinner and the person who is driving has had a few too many. The driver, although drunk, in-
sists on driving home and won't give up the car keys."

What would you do? _____
How would you get home? _____
Would you let your friend drive? _____
Why or why not? _____
What would you say to your friend the next day?_____

_____

SITUATION 4 (Child reads to parents)
"You are at a social gathering, talking to a group of people.
One person starts to tell a dirty joke that offends you. You
feel uncomfortable and don't want to listen to those kinds
of jokes."

How could you express your thoughts and feelings assertively? _____
What if everyone else wants to hear the joke? _____

_____

What if others tease you or call you a spoilsport? _____

_____

Exercise 6   **PARENT and CHILD**

THE WORLD AROUND YOU

Every day you hear examples of each of the communication styles: at the store, on television, in school, in your own conversations, virtually anywhere that people communicate with one another. Pay attention to those styles so you can learn to recognize them in others as well as in yourself.

When you and your child are together, point out the styles you hear. "She was pretty passive when that guy cut in front of her in line." "The actor in that show was aggressive when he demanded his own way." See how quickly each of you can spot the styles and point them out to each other.

Parents who have a sophisticated grasp of communciation can sometimes, in their zeal, become manipulative. If you are presenting yourself in a manner calculated to invoke a certain response from your teen, you will never give your teen a clear message. Your teen will learn to do the same, and you will both end up being actors in an artificial relationship instead of two people who should really know one another.

If you want your teen to be assertive and honest, you must be so yourself.

4

FITTING IN

"Aw gee, Mom. All the kids are doing it. I don't see why I can't. You're ruining my life!"—Pressured teenager

Sound familiar? At a certain age, all young people want to be just like their friends. They want to look the same, talk the same, walk the same, think the same. Parents usually find this drive for teenage conformity merely frustrating or amusing. We don't worry too much and may even recognize this drive for what it is—a young person learning to "fit in," to avoid deviation from a society to which he or she belongs.

All their lives our children have been taught to follow norms, to be like other people who live the right kind of lives. We set norms in our homes that we expect children to follow. We help enforce the norms of their schools and churches. And often we have helped them identify the norms of their friends and peers:

"Why don't you keep your room clean like Joey?"
"Look, all your friends can ride their bikes without training wheels. You can too."
"Sarah just had a big birthday party with twenty friends over. Would you like to have a big party for your birthday too?"

Fitting in is what helps us to be enough like our neighbors so that we have a common ground of fraternity. It holds our families, our communities, even our country together. But fitting in can be carried too far. A group of teens may wear the same unattractive haircut and listen to the same rock star or flock to the same movie.

While parents may find these behaviors distasteful, teens usually pass through these fads unscathed. What happens when taking drugs becomes the "thing to do" or when engaging in sex becomes a rite of passage? What if the popular crowd likes to get drunk? This is when attempts to fit in may jeopardize a teen's health and future.

Picture a setting sometimes used in films about young people. A small group of teenage boys and girls get together for a light-hearted evening. Pizza, soda, popcorn. "We'll play some cards," one of the boys suggests. As a few lucky card players win some rounds, the stakes get higher. Someone suggests with a smirk, "Why don't we play strip poker? Come on, you're not chickens are you?" Afraid to admit embarrassment, the group is silent. One boy, or girl for that matter, trying to present a facade of coolness and sophistication, agrees with the idea and says, "If any of you are babies about these things, just leave now."

And so the highly charged card session begins. Most of the members of the group don't really feel comfortable with the situation, but they feel powerless to stop it. In fact, they even challenge someone who does try to stop the game. In a few short minutes, seven or eight teens have been pressured into doing something they probably did not want to do. They are victims of peer pressure.

Studies have shown that young people who begin to abuse drugs do so frequently because of peer pressure. A group of friends will generally practice the same pattern of drug use; the same for smoking or drinking. Whether or not a teen has sex may also depend on peer pressure. Although sexual urges are developing in the physically maturing adolescent, it is generally not the biological drive alone that leads to intercourse. Consider the boy who feels his virginity is both obvious and shameful, or the girl who is given an ultimatum by a boy she really likes: sex or a breakup.

Peer pressure is a powerful force. Of course, peer pressure may not be direct; it may not even be real. But as long as teens PERCEIVE an expectation among people their age, then they will respond accordingly. This is often referred to as "perceived pressure." No one is pushing the young person to do something; no one is daring or teasing him.

The perceived pressure arises from the teen's internal discomfort over an anticipated judgment by peers. Thus, the image parents may hold of a drug pusher victimizing sons is not wholly accurate, nor is the image of a teenage gigolo suavely seducing daughters. While pushers and gigolos are not unheard of, they are rarely the major factor in a teen's decision to use drugs, drink, or engage in sex. As difficult as it is to acknowledge, parents must recognize an element of free will in the actions of their children.

As adults we CAN empathize with young people. We were teens once and no doubt felt pressures to act a certain way. Moreover, we are still prey to peer pressure. "What will the neighbors think" may still provide a standard for some of us. We dress as many of our colleagues at work dress. We bite our tongues to keep us from telling an anecdote that is inappropriate for the group we are with. We feel compelled to invite the Smiths to dinner because they invited us to their last two social events. We may want our kids to join the same club or team as the other kids of parents in our social circle. Whether we are aware of it or not, we are often faced with peer pressure—and we find the pressure hard to resist even as adults. Ask yourself some of the following questions about social pressures:

- Have you ever put in many extra hours on the job just because your co-workers did and you felt you had to put up a show?
- Have you ever exaggerated achievements of your own or another member of your family during a conversation with boastful friends?
- Have you ever accepted a drink you didn't want just because your host at a cocktail party pressed you to take one?
- Can you think of any other situations in which you did something only because you thought it was expected of you?

Who is a Likely Victim of Peer Pressure?

No one is immune from peer pressure; some individuals, however, are better able to cope with peer pressure situations than others. Which teens are most susceptible to influences from peers? Below are key characteristics, some that may from time to time apply to all teens and some that apply to only a few teens.

High Risk Signals

New Situations in which a teen feels insecure. An example is the youngster who graduates from grade school to junior high school or from junior high to senior high school. These transition times can be stressful, especially if they involve making new friends or fitting in with new peer groups.

Instability that suddenly occurs in the teen's secure and stable environment. An example is the child whose parents are going through separation or divorce, or the child who has moved to a new city and must make new friends.

Lack of skills to resist peer pressure can lead teens into traps. Does your teen know how to say NO in an assertive but socially acceptable way that maintains friendships and self-esteem?

Feeling sad can cause some teens to try risk-taking behaviors, especially if the young person has very little family support or has only limited perspective on the temporary nature of feeling sad.

Uncertain value systems can confuse a teen, leading to more experimentation or improper behaviors. An example is the youngster whose parents engage in certain behaviors while telling children to "Do as I say, not as I do." Another example may be the youngster who has not been given the opportunity to explore her own values in discussions with parents.

Rebelliousness can lead some sons and daughters to choose actions that run in opposition to parents' beliefs. Sometimes the rebellion is designed to get attention, establish independence, or express anger and hostility.

Low self-esteem can stand in the way of a teen developing his own personal set of values. The teen who doesn't feel good about himself often tries too hard to convince peers that he is mature by showing off or taking risks.

Extreme loneliness or lack of the social skills needed to make friends can lead a pained youngster to go to almost any length to gain acceptance.

Helping Teens Resist Peer Pressure

You CAN help your teen determine the limits of healthy conformity and resist potentially harmful pressure from peers. The process takes time and a light touch. Communication is an essential tool, as is imagining yourself in your teen's position, having your teen's immature social skills.

Even though a teen's peers assume a greater role of influence than ever before, you as a parent still retain strong influence. The key is to make the most of the impact you have on your son or daughter. Your impact will be greater if you acknowledge and respect your teen's independence in certain areas of his life and treat him as a maturing, changing teen and not as a child or as an adult.

Here are several strategies that can give your child the ability to be true to himself.

Practice Saying NO in a Tough Spot

It's such a simple word, but we all have difficulty saying NO sometimes. You may shake your head and wonder how at two years of age your child's favorite word was NO, but how a dozen years later your teen seems unable to use that simple word among friends. As a parent who taught that two-year-old to become agreeable, you have a responsibility to teach your teen to become more independent.

We all assume that young people know how to say NO, but really they don't, especially in situations where they perceive pressure or critical judgement from peers. A list of "Ways to Refuse" appears on page 48; it is followed by an exercise to help you practice these strategies. We recommend that you and your child complete the exercise for the following reasons:

- Your child can actively practice saying NO.
- You can be an effective role model in demonstrating ways to resist pressure.
- You and your child can think of better answers as a team than you can individually.
- Your child will be better prepared in the event that he or she has to face similar situations later.

After you have done the exercise, continue to practice periodically to reinforce your child's skill in saying NO in difficult pressure situations.

WAYS TO REFUSE

The following list gives examples of different ways to refuse a sexual advance or a drug offer. Read the list aloud to learn the different techniques.

Strategy

Pressure	Response
	Simple "No"
Do you want a beer?	"No, thanks." or "No."
	Emphatic "No"
Don't be a chicken.	"No, I *don't* want to do that!"
	Repetitive "No"
Let's go smoke pot. Come on. No one's home. We won't get caught.	"No." "No." "No."
	Turn the Tables
If you really loved me you'd let me touch you.	"If you loved me you wouldn't insist."
	Give a Reason
Want a cigarette?	"No, I don't smoke. The smell stays in my hair and clothes."
	Ignore the Person
Don't be a jerk. It's only pot. Try some.	Simply ignore the pressure and don't say a word.
	Leave the Scene
Hey, everyone else is pairing up. Want to go to the bedroom with me?	Walk out of there.

Steer Clear of the Situation

If you know there will be drugs at a party, don't go. If you suspect someone may try to pressure you to have sex, don't go out with that person.

Call in the Cavalry

If someone tries to touch you and you don't like it, or tries to make you do anything you don't want, tell them to stop and threaten to tell someone with authority (e.g., parents, teacher, police).

Rise Above the Pressure

Why don't you want to try marijuana? Everyone's doing it.	"I don't need that stuff and I don't need to be like everyone else."

Exercise 7   **PARENT and CHILD**

WHAT COULD YOU DO IF...?

Some methods for saying NO work better than others depending on the situation. Below are some pressure situations that preteens and teenagers face. Review the "Ways to Refuse" with your child (page 48) and ask which method(s) could be used in each situation. Write the method(s) in the blank next to the statement.

What Could You Do If...

Preteens

1. A friend offers you a puff on a cigarette? _____
_____

2. You walk home from school and pass by a park every day where teenagers are drinking. They call out to you, "Hey kid, come join us." _____

3. A stranger asks you to get into his car to give him directions? _____

4. Your best friend's parents are gone and he or she wants you to drink some of their liquor? _____

5. A group of kids are trying pot and they call you a "chicken" because you won't do it with them? _____
_____

6. An adult touches you in a place that makes you feel strange? _____

7. A friend offers you a cigarette and, when you refuse, he keeps saying "Why not?" _____

8. Someone in your class dares you to smoke pot? _____
_____

(continued)

(*Exercise 7 continued*)

Teenagers

1. Your best friend wants to try marijuana and asks you to try it too? _____

_____

2. Someone who has a reputation for being "fast," or very sexual, wants to go out with you? You suspect that person will try to pressure you to have sex. _____

_____

3. On the way to the football game, your friends open a six-pack of beer and call you a baby for refusing to drink?

_____

4. After the movies, your date asks for a kiss and you'd rather not kiss this person? _____

_____

5. Even though you've refused nicely, your date tries to pressure you for a kiss and won't ease up until you do?

_____

6. A classmate invites you to a party you'd really like to go to and says, "My parents are gone, so there will be booze and pot"? _____

_____

7. You're with a friend on the way to the school dance. Your friend is drinking and keeps bugging you to drink as well?

_____

8. You've started hanging around with a new group of friends and you want them to like you. In the bathroom at school they light up a cigarette and pass it around to you?

Foster Independent Thinking

The world is filled with interesting puzzles and questions. Ask your teen what she thinks about issues not related to hot topics such as drugs and sex. For example, do you know what she thinks about education, the value of a life, capital punishment, our political future, war, happiness, the degree of control we have over our lives? Remember, however, to ask her opinions as you would a respected adult.

As a parent, you can too easily fall into the temptation of pointing out faulty reasoning, trying to browbeat your child into your way of thinking, passing judgment, or debating an issue. If you don't agree with the thoughts of your son or daughter, let it be. Simply state your views and let your teen know that you respect his or her opinion. After all, the goal is to raise a healthy, independent adult, not a stifled clone of yourself.

DOs and DON'Ts of Talking to Your Teen

DO	DON'T
Encourage frank discussion	Be threatened by a difference of opinion
Respect your teen's privacy	Pry or ask embarrassing questions
Praise independent thinking	Insist on agreement
Let teens make some of their own decisions	Judge too critically
Let teens help set rules	Lecture or argue
Ask your child's opinions often	Listen only halfway

Explore What "Really Is"

How often have you heard that "all the kids are doing it"? The plea is not just a ploy on the part of your teen; he really does believe that nearly everyone but him can stay up late, go to the game on Saturday, have a custom-made bicycle, and so on. Likewise, he may believe that nearly every other kid his age is smoking dope or drinking beer before the dance.

The feeling that "everyone is doing something but me" is an uncomfortable one, especially for the teen who wants so much to fit in and be part of the crowd. The irony is that NOT everyone is doing it. Not every teen on the block drinks beer. Not every popular girl has gone "all the way." Not every boy in junior high school smokes. Thus, the pressure to do something in order to fit in can be just a perceived pressure, not a real one.

You can help counter your teen's claims, but you will need to do your homework. How many boys on the block have custom-made bicycles? How many do not? How many of the community's teens show up drunk at dances? Keep in mind that while many youngsters may have TRIED marijuana or cigarettes, very few use these substances regularly, and many who say they have had sex are really making untrue boasts. Knowing that she is not alone can give a big boost to the teen who feels pressure to have sex, take drugs, or drink, yet who isn't sure she really wants to or else has the nagging feeling that such behaviors are wrong.

In exploring what really is, make certain you get to know more about the people who influence your child. Find out who your child admires and wants to be like. Take time to talk to his friends. Ask what other teens in the community think or do. As a parent, you must widen your range of exposure to the norms in your son's or daughter's peer group.

Building Self-Esteem

Consider how differently you respond to pressures or make decisions when you feel good about yourself than when you don't feel so good about who you are. Because they are at an age where they are groping for identity, self-confidence, and independence, teens can be especially vulnerable to making poor decisions or responding without thinking. Families are very important in the process of discovering "who am I?" and "what value do I have?" Parents have a definite responsibility for the way a teen feels about himself. Chapter 2—"How to Talk to Your Child"—can give you useful tips on how to build your child's self-esteem. (See the section entitled "Encourage.")

Explore Fears about Saying NO

"Dare to be different." The statement sums up pretty well the courage it sometimes takes to resist conformity. Have frank discussions with your teen about what it means to resist the currently fashionable teen behaviors, especially behaviors such as drug taking, drinking, or sex. What would REALLY happen if your son said NO to drinking at a party? What would REALLY happen if your daughter said NO to the advances of her favorite boyfriend?

Sometimes teens have unrealistic fears of what they might lose by choosing to say NO or to be different. Perhaps the consequence most feared by teens is the loss of a friend or friends. First discuss how likely it would be for a friend to be lost so easily. Then spend some time defining a true friend, one who is worth having as a friend. Exercises 8, 9, and 10 can help clarify the values and definitions of friendship.

Exercise 8   **PARENT and CHILD**

WHAT MAKES A GOOD FRIEND?

We consider some people our acquaintances, some people our friends, and some very special people our good friends. Why are they different? Who do we feel the closest to, confide in, spend time with, and listen to the most?

Good friends are important, and they can influence us a lot. Think of three qualities or characteristics a good friend should have and write them in the spaces below without looking at each other's answers:

Parent: 1. _____

           2. _____

           3. _____

Child: 1. _____

           2. _____

           3. _____

Were any of your answers the same? _____

_____

Do you agree with each other's answers, or do you look for different things in a friend? _____

_____

On the next page are several statements about friendships. Read them aloud together. Think silently about each statement and decide if it's true or false. Take turns at being first to give your answer.

If you both agree that a statement is true, check the "TRUE" column. If you both agree it is false, check the "FALSE" column. If you disagree with each other, check the "CAN'T DECIDE" column.

It is okay to disagree: the statements may be interpreted in different ways or you may have different values about friendships. The point of this exercise is to learn the values each of you hold and to examine those values.

(continued)

(Exercise 8 continued)

	TRUE	FALSE	CAN'T DECIDE
1. A friend should always stand up for you, even if you have done something wrong.			
2. Friends can influence the way you act and the choices you make.			
3. If my friend were doing something that was bad for him or her, I would tell my friend to stop.			
4. It is okay to lie to protect a friend.			
5. I can disagree with my friend without losing that friendship.			
6. A good friend should never ask me to do something that would get me in trouble.			
7. Everyone needs friendships.			
8. Sometimes being a good friend might mean telling on a friend when he or she has done something really bad.			
9. I could say NO to a friend who offered me something I didn't want, like alcohol or drugs.			
10. A good friend would not pressure me to do something I really didn't want to do.			
11. I would lend money to a friend.			
12. Friends should always be there when you need them.			
13. It is important that my family accept the friends I choose.			
14. Sometimes you may have to hurt a friend.			
15. A friend always has my best interests at heart.			

Exercise 9   **PARENT and CHILD**

FRIENDSHIP DILEMMAS

Sometimes even the best of friendships experience conflicts. Below are three different "Friendship Dilemmas," one for preteens, one for teenagers, and one for adults. Take turns reading aloud the dilemma for your age group and then tell what you would do in that situation.

PRETEEN: You spent a lot of time on your homework last night and thought up some really creative answers. Your best friend went out to dinner with his/her parents and didn't get home in time to finish the homework. Your friend asks to copy your homework, but you are afraid the teacher will find out and give you an "F." On the other hand, your friend isn't doing well in the class and will surely get an "F" for having no homework. What would you say to your friend and why?

TEENAGER: Your friend has invited you to a movie Saturday night to celebrate your birthday. You've been waiting a long time to see the movie with your friend, and you've both been talking about it a lot. On Saturday afternoon, your friend is given one ticket to a concert with a really popular band that same night. The concert has been sold out for months, so you can't get a ticket. Your friend leaves you a note telling you that s/he is going to the concert tonight and not to the movie. What would you say to your friend and why?

ADULT: You have just bought a brand new car. Your insurance is still being arranged, and you are the only one covered for now. You have told everyone in your family that no one but you is to drive the car until it is fully insured. Your good friend calls and says she must pick up her child across town right away; she asks to borrow your car. You cannot drive your friend yourself right now and you don't want to lend her your car. What would you say to your friend and why?

Discuss the following questions:

- Do you agree or disagree with each other's answers? Why or why not?

- Would you have done or said the same thing? If not, what might you have done instead?

Exercise 10   **PARENT and CHILD**

LOOKING AT YOUR OWN FRIENDSHIPS

Write down the name(s) of your best friend(s):

Parent: _____

_____

Child: _____

_____

Think about the things you value in best friends, the things you would do for them, the things you expect them to do for you, the characteristics you've just thought about in the preceding exercises.

Then discuss your answers to the following questions with each other:

1. Do the friends you have now live up to your expectations of what a good friend should be? (Why or why not?)

2. If you decided that one of your friends no longer acted the way you thought a good friend should act, what would you do?

5

MEDIA MANIA

By the time a young person graduates from high school, he or she has spent more time watching television than attending school.

Let's be honest with ourselves. Why do we read books or watch television? For entertainment, of course, but that isn't the only reason we engross ourselves in movies, TV shows, radio programs, magazines, newspapers, books, and other forms of media.

While many of us do not care to admit it, we learn a lot from the media. What we know about the world outside our communities, what we think about our society as a whole, and how we perceive the lifestyles of people very different from ourselves have all been shaped in part by what we have seen or heard from our "entertainment sources."

There is nothing inherently wrong in learning from the media. Some TV shows, for example, have provided us with models of excellent parents, perhaps ones we try to follow when confronted with a difficult situation. You may have felt validated by seeing one of TV's perfect parents or spouses take the same action you did to solve a particular problem. On the other hand, you may have tried to avoid acting like one of the TV characters who ended up creating more problems than he or she solved.

The media also provide common grounds for communicating with others. We talk about last night's TV shows or events that happen in the news. We use common media figures as part of our communications—"He's just like Archie Bunker"—and media slogans as everyday expressions—"You deserve a break today."

We take in and use media messages daily on a conscious level, using all forms of media to gain information, form opinions, and communicate with others.

Media and the Unconscious Mind

The media can also influence us unconsciously, or without our active acceptance of the messages portrayed. We form very subtle associations between the media and different thoughts, feelings, and attitudes. Have you ever found yourself buying a particular brand of a product just because you heard it advertised recently? Do certain radio jingles for products go through your mind after you hear them, even though you don't want to think about them? Maybe you even hum them without realizing it.

Our concepts of what is "right" or "good" or "socially acceptable" can be subtly influenced by the media without our conscious acceptance of these values. For example, many people judge women against concepts portrayed in magazines, on TV, and in movies. To meet these standards, a woman must be ultra thin and beautiful. This value persists even though the overwhelming majority of women aren't ultra thin. The strength of this media message is evidenced by the fact that over 80% of women periodically put themselves on weight-reduction diets.

The media may promote a certain political candidate to be "trustworthy, honest, and experienced" and we may vote for that candidate simply because he is a familiar face, even if we know nothing about the issues he supports or his actual qualities. Similarly, we may distrust another candidate whom the media links with a scandal, even if the report is later found to be untrue.

The media can make strong, lasting impressions on us without our even being aware of it. Has a certain song ever brought you back to an earlier time in your life and evoked vivid memories of what was happening then? At the time you heard that song, you may not have realized that it would stay with you so long. Do you remember slogans from products advertised when you were much younger? "Mmmmm good, mmmmm good," "I'd walk a mile for a . . . ," "A little dab'll do ya'," "I'd rather fight than switch." How about theme songs from different TV shows?

Would you recognize the show by the song, even though it's been 15 years since you've seen it?

The conscious and unconscious messages we pick up from the media can be long-lasting and influence our attitudes and our actions. Even as adults we can be subtly influenced. We can, however, moderate that influence and select what makes sense because we are experienced enough to be able to make our own judgments about the truths or fictions we witness through the media.

The Young Are Easily Influenced

What about youngsters who have less experience on which to base judgments about the validity of what they see and hear in the media? Do they view the media as a window on the world?

At a very superficial level, we can detect obvious influence from celebrities. Adolescents often dress to look like a popular rock star or TV personality. Younger children may plead for items they see frequently advertised on TV or on cereal boxes. It is harder to identify the more subtle, unconscious influences on value systems or life perspectives.

> Dean came through the kitchen on his way out for the evening. His hair was slicked back with a peroxide-lightened forelock, shaved close at the sides then spilling over from the top like a spider plant. His tight trousers were covered by a long, loose shirt—very wrinkled, of course. But his parents could live with that. It was the half scowl etched on his lips, the posture that looked like he was about to attack someone that worried them. They knew Dean had adopted the popular dress style of the current teen idols. What they did not know, but feared, was that he might have the same sense of futility and recklessness echoed throughout so many of the rock songs he and his friends listened to.

Many experts have noted the degree of violence to which TV viewers are exposed and raised questions about the hazards of exposing young people to that violence. Those involved with drug abuse prevention likewise fear the effects on youngsters who watch the glamorized lives of drug-takers and drinkers. They point to the influence of popular songs about getting high and advertisements showing romanticized scenes involving alcohol. On television alone, alcohol manufacturers spend $370 million a year on advertising. The tobacco industry spends $690 million a year on advertising in the nonbroadcast media. You can bet that they wouldn't spend so much money on advertising if they didn't think it would increase sales.

There are fewer statistics on the amount of sex shown in the media. A recent study, however, indicated that the average television viewer will be exposed to 9,000 sex scenes in a year's viewing. Unfortunately, many of those scenes will not only involve sex, but often sex that is abusive or deviant—the stuff of titillating entertainment appeal. Of course, the use of sexuality is a well-known tool in the advertising business. A brief scan of the advertising in magazines or on television will certainly bear that out.

What are the messages your child is receiving from the media? Try the exercises on the following pages. Exercise 11 is for you alone; Exercises 12 and 13 are for you and your child to explore together. The exercises will provide you with insight into your child's world of media influences. Be careful not to jump to hasty conclusions, because the message you see may be inconsequential to your child. For example, your teen may listen to a song not because the lyrics are about drugs, but because the beat is good or because the performers are popular with his peers. Your youngster may watch a favorite TV program not for the hinted sexuality, but because the plot is genuinely adventuresome and interesting.

Nonetheless, even these indirect messages can engrave an image in your youngster's mind. The point is that you should be aware, not alarmed or reactionary.

Negative Consequences Are Often Ignored

Admittedly, the media often does portray the negative consequences of drug use or illicit sex. The question is how attuned the viewer may be to that message. Some experts wonder if young people, given their focus on the immediate here and now, may not just pay attention to the excitement of the action-packed moment rather than the more delayed future consequences of

KIDS, DRUGS, AND SEX

IT'S PRIME TIME, DO YOU KNOW
WHAT YOUR CHILDREN ARE WATCHING?

What do you know about the characters your child looks up to? What about the songs he sings to himself? Do you know what is so appealing in the plot of that short story she has been reading?

Explore the answers to the following questions. You will probably have to watch your child's favorite TV programs, listen to his favorite songs, and skim some of her favorite reading materials.

- What TV programs does your child watch regularly?
  Who are the lead characters?
  Describe the ways they look (dress, cleanliness, posture, facial
    expressions).

  Describe the ways they act (aloof and superior or friendly and kind;
    smoker, drinker, or "clean"; reckless or cautious; taunting in sex-
    uality or modest and appropriate in sexual behaviors).
  What is the lead character's outlook on life?

- What are your child's favorite songs?
  Describe what the songs are about.
  Decide if the songs portray a general happiness about life.

- What films has your child been impressed with recently?
  Outline the plots.
  Characterize the hero or heroine of the films.
  To what extent do drugs or sex play a major part in this film?

- What does your child read?
  State the theme of the book/story/article.
  Characterize the individuals described in the writing.

Now think about all the messages you have just explored.

What is the general message about drugs, drinking, and sexuality?

What are the negative consequences portrayed?

What about the positive consequences (excitement, wealth, glamour, relief from worries or problems, being with a fast or "in" crowd)?

wrong-doing, consequences to which teens often feel immune. Seeing only part of what is going on is called selective perception. We all edit out certain items we do not understand or do not want to see or hear. It's natural.

In other words, teens may find the sexual scenes in films and ads too stimulating to consider that they are witnessing only part of the real picture. They do not watch the arousing scene thinking about the potential consequences: unwanted pregnancy or a sexually transmitted disease, a relationship that gets too heavy too fast and becomes difficult to escape, a trap of not being able to say NO since YES has been said once already.

Likewise, the glamor of drinking or getting high may mask the harder realities: the beer drinker at the party ending up in a pile of automotive metal wrapped around a tree; the cocaine user finding his addiction leading to far more depression that euphoria; the drug experimenter winding up with a law enforcement record that wrecks his future hopes of education or job; the "good-time Charlie" who gets into a fight, losing a front tooth and some good friends.

With a little involvement, you can help your child be a more sophisticated media user. Let's face it, the media is an important part of our lives. We can't ban everything we find distasteful, and we can't moderate our children's media habits forever. Therefore, it is up to us to teach them how to use the media well and how to think about the things they see, read, and hear. You can teach your child to *actively* examine media messages rather than to *passively* accept them.

Working Together

Listening to music, watching television, or going to the movies can be enjoyable family entertainment. With a little effort, they can also be educational and provide you with the opportunity to influence your child's media habits and her opinions about the things she sees or hears. If you participate in your child's media entertainment time, you have the opportunity to express your thoughts concerning situations that you are both viewing or reading.

In chapter 2, you learned that direct questioning or confronta-

Exercise 12 **PARENT and CHILD**

TALLY THE TAUNTS

Just how many scenes on television or in magazines involve the use of sex to get your attention? Sex is used to sell products, even those that have nothing to do with sex appeal. It is used to tease you into watching certain programs.

For this exercise, pick out two evenings to watch prime-time television. As you watch the programs, keep a tally of all the sexually stimulating scenes you see both in commercials and during the shows. Sexually stimulating scenes can involve not only the sex act, but also a suggestive look or conversation, a sexy body, close hugs, or any item that brings to mind something to do with sex.

Hours of viewing: _____

	During TV shows	*In a commercial*
Number of sex scenes:	_____	_____

Many people are surprised by the number of taunts they find on TV. Were you? What kind of message might someone get from these sexually stimulating scenes?

_____

_____

Now try the same exercise by looking through two magazines. Pick two magazines that are different from each other, for example, a teen magazine and a car magazine.

#1 magazine title: _____

Number of sexual scenes, written
  or depicted: _____

#2 magazine title: _____

Number of sexual scenes, written
  or depicted: _____

For further discussion:
Were the sexually stimulating scenes you found on TV or in the magazine really necessary to the main plot of the story or for selling the product?

If there were instances in which the scenes were not entirely relevant or could have been eliminated, discuss why the scenes were used.

COMMERCIAL COUNT

Advertising is the most blatant form of influence. Often the advertiser, in trying to sell a product, is also conveying a subtle image that supposedly comes with the product. The five S's describe the more commonly used techniques:

Sex appeal
Status (wealth, prestige)
Sociability (fun, friends)
Strength (power, machismo)
Smarts (for choosing the best)

Spend a couple of evenings during your family's favorite TV viewing time to survey what the commercials are selling and how they are selling it. Place check marks in the columns. You can also use this exercise to examine magazine ads.

HOURS OF VIEWING _____

PRODUCT   TECHNIQUE

ALCOHOL	MEDICINES	SEX	STATUS	SOCIABILITY	STRENGTH	SMARTS
Example: Brand X beer		✔		✔	✔	

(continued)

(*Exercise 13 continued*)

Sum up the messages the commercials are conveying to your family.

_____

_____

_____

_____

Discuss ways your children can be smart consumers and be more critical of the advertising they see. For example, what information was left out about the product? (Drinking can make you sick, fat, or careless; taking headache pills can mask a more serious problem or get you into the habit of relying on "magic pills"; jeans do not make the wearer more personable or attractive.)

_____

_____

_____

_____

Does the technique used really have something to do with the product being advertised?

_____

_____

_____

_____

tion can often make your teen defensive. If you focus on an outside character, however, you may be more likely to open a discussion about difficult topics. Consider the following example:

Pete overheard his son talking about a new movie he had seen with his friends. The movie was one of those popular comedies about a group of teenage friends—not the type a father would really enjoy. Pete listened to the boys joking about a few of the scenes and realized it had been a long time since he and his son had joked just as the boys were doing now. In fact it had been at least a year and a half since they had gone to a movie together.

Pete decided to go to the movie himself and see just what his son was viewing. He almost enjoyed the story, but, more importantly, he began to get an idea of how teenage boys were portrayed on the screen. He wanted to talk to his son about a few of the scenes he found disturbing, particularly ones involving drunken antics and irresponsible sex.

Knowing that his son would tune him out if he began to critique the film, Pete instead related one of the more humorous scenes to the family during dinner. As he began to tell the story, his son contributed additional information that Pete had left out. Together they told their family about a few more funny incidents in the movie. Over the next couple of days, Pete and his son would occasionally mention something that happened in the film. They acted as though they shared an "inside joke."

One evening soon after Pete had gone to the movie, he saw his son watching TV alone. Pete sat down and watched too. The TV program was about a detective, but one subplot featured a man pursuing the affections of an attractive woman. "Boy, he sure knows how to attract a woman. I was thinking . . . those guys in the movie we saw probably wouldn't stand a chance with a girl the way they were acting," Pete said offhandedly to his son. His son did not say anything, so Pete continued. "I don't think that women, or girls for that matter, in this day and age really like being pushed around. Just think about your sister and her friends. Could you imagine that they would want a boy to bully them?" His son answered, "Beth would probably kick the rear end of any guy that gave her a hard time. She gives me a hard enough time and I'm just her brother. I'd hate to be a guy going out with her on a date." Pete and his son continued talking for about 15 minutes, discussing respect for girls and how the tough guy image in the movies was off the mark. They even spent a couple of minutes beginning to explore what girls thought about having sex. The conversation did not last long, but Pete knew that the next time they might talk in more depth about sexuality, so he did not push his son into sharing more of his thoughts on intimacy.

Pete and his son also made plans to go to see the new adventure movie showing at the theatre downtown—Dad would even pick up the tab.

Pete used the opportunity at hand and paved the way for a new one. You have opportunities too. From a TV show about teenage rape or pregnancy you may discuss what other responses the TV character may have tried or what precautions could have prevented the problem in the first place. From a newspaper article about the high rate of teen drinking and related car accidents you could ask your teen if the statistics seem accurate according to his impression of the community. Ask your teen what he thinks may be successful strategies for preventing the dangers of drinking and driving.

Nearly any story about people involves social pressures to conform. Try using such a story to help your child recognize pressures from peers and think for herself. How could a character have stood his ground and said NO to pressures from peers? What ways would have allowed him to still keep his friends and even gain their respect? Rewrite the storyline in your imaginations so that the end turns out differently.

Take an active role in shaping your family's media habits. There are many good television programs, songs, books, and films. Some of these even try to provide guidance on living successfully and happily. Encourage the enjoyment of these enriching media messages.

In order to discourage your family from partaking of particularly negative media programs, try finding alternative ac-

Exercise 14   **PARENT and CHILD**

ARCHAEOLOGISTS' SURVEY

Here is an exercise for you and your child to do together. In working through this exercise, try to forget who you are now and what you think about today's society—you are going to be transported more than a hundred years into the future.

Imagine that it is the year 2100 A.D. You are archaeologists trying to learn more about the culture of the late 1900s. Luckily, you have discovered a large warehouse of record albums, video cassettes of TV programs, reels of movie films, the best selling books, and the popular magazines of the period.

As you review each of your media treasures, what do you begin to see as the way the society was portrayed? Give specific examples from the different types of media. (In considering TV, for example, do you find that the police programs show a society filled with criminals or with law-abiding citizens? Are the youngsters on TV innocent or wise beyond their age? Are grandparents revered or ridiculed? Do the shows take place in the society at the time or are they more escapist, such as Westerns and science fiction?)

What do the films, books, TV programs, and songs say about the young adolescent living at the time?

Now try to guess how the culture of 2100 A.D. was shaped by the culture of the 1980s. Were there any lasting effects? Did people learn anything about themselves? Did they try to change?

tivities such as going to concerts or sports events, pitching in to make a fabulous dessert, going to the pool, taking the dog for a pleasant stroll. Sometimes you may have to take a firm stance and insist that a program not be seen or a story not be read. Such a drastic measure, however, is best saved as a last resort. Censorship often backfires, making the forbidden program or book all the more enticing. Just remember what happened during Prohibition—people continued to drink, but they hid their drinking and became further removed from any type of control.

Our American society has long complained about the negative effects of the media. But the media will be negative only if we allow it to be. While we may have limited personal power to change TV programming or news reporting habits, we can turn current media content to our advantage—by talking and by sharing what we feel and fear. What we tend to forget is that WE too are part of the media, for we are the audience. Do not let your family be part of a victimized, passive audience. Play an active role.

6

DO YOU SEE WHAT I SEE?

What is a parent? A role model, a nurturer, a protector, and an ally. Being a parent is a very special job. Take pride in that job, for it is one of the most important roles you will ever undertake.

Follow My Lead: Parent as Role Model

Kids, drugs, and sex—that is the problem you want to deal with. But in combatting it you also need to look at parents, drugs, and sex—in other words, you, drugs, and sex. To expect young people to practice certain behaviors and to act on specific values is asking a lot if they have no role model.

When you became a parent, you acquired many responsibilities—feeding, sheltering, safeguarding, and nurturing your children. But you also became a role model. As part of that responsibility, you need to examine your own behaviors and the messages they convey about substance abuse and sex. Research shows that parents' behaviors are good predictors of how a child will act.

Being a good role model in regard to drinking, for example, means no drinking and driving, not drinking too much, not using alcohol as a crutch, and saying NO instead of always saying YES to offers of a drink.

If the message you want to convey to your child is "Make good decisions about sex," then be a good role model. Avoid off-color jokes, sexist comments, loose responses to others of the opposite sex (which may be innocent but misinterpreted), a focus on the physical attributes of members of the opposite sex, and so on.

Exercise 15 will help you evaluate the kind of role model you are to your child.

Exercise 15   **PARENT**

LOOK AT YOURSELF

How do you see your role as a parent? Take this brief test right now to gauge your attitudes. Read each statement. If you agree with the statement circle the number next to it. If you disagree with it, leave it blank.

1. I always set a good example for my children.

2. I expect my children to do as I do.

3. I try to set a good example but have developed some bad habits that I have not had the strength to break.

4. I try to set a good example but sometimes my children must overlook my behaviors and do the opposite of what I do.

5. I have some bad habits but I am an adult and can make decisions about my behavior based on weighing the consequences.

6. My children do not have enough life experience to make decisions about behaviors that will affect their lives— they must rely on me to tell them how to live right.

7. I have told my children to "do as I say, not as I do."

8. My children must respect their elders.

9. My teenager can make his own decisions about what behaviors are appropriate.

10. I have never behaved in a way that I would not want my children to imitate.

11. My youngsters are at the age when they have made it clear that they do not plan to be like their parents, so it makes little difference what I do.

(continued)

(*Exercise 15 continued*)

Response Key

If you agreed with numbers

1, 2, 10:   Let us know who you are. We ourselves have always wanted to find the perfect person to emulate.

5, 6, 7, 8:   Question whether you may be too controlling. If you answered yes to 5 and 7, you are not expecting enough of yourself—try to improve your own behaviors. If you answered yes to 6 and 8, you may not be letting your children grow up to be mature adults.

3, 4:   Good for you for having an honest view of yourself. Try harder to live the way you would want your children to follow.

9, 11:   Ask yourself if you have given up your role as leader. Young people need more guidance than you may be providing. If you agreed with 9 then it's wonderful that you have such trust and such a terrific teen—just avoid the denial syndrome.

What about those families in which a parent may be a heavy smoker or drinker yet the children abstain? That does of course happen, for young people learn from their parents' mistakes. A parent handicapped by emphysema, cancer, or alcoholism gives a strong message about the negative consequences of such behaviors. But that seems too high a price to pay just to say to your children, "See what can happen?"

On the flip side, what about those families in which a parent may be a non-smoker and a very moderate and sensible drinker yet the children sneak cigarettes and go on drinking binges? That too can happen and the reasons can be very complex, as you have been learning from this book.

But these issues do not undermine the importance of good parental role models. Having good role models does not guarantee faultless adolescent behavior but it certainly increases the odds that the young person will hold to his family's values.

Being a role model is a responsibility some parents take less seriously than more basic responsibilities, such as providing an income to the family or keeping a clean home. They may begin parenthood realizing that their sweet little baby learns how to walk, talk, and eat by imitating their actions. Yet as their child grows older, they misinterpret her growing independence and personal decision making as a sign that she no longer needs examples to imitate. Moreover, they see that the behaviors that their child does imitate are generally those of young peers.

It is true that as a youngster enters adolescence, he tends to find influence among a wider circle of role models, such as school chums or celebrity idols. But sharing the spotlight with other in fluencing persons does not mean that you as a parent are left with no influence. It does mean, however, that you may need to make sure that the values and behaviors you are trying to instill in your child are clearly and directly communicated.

ACTIONS SPEAK LOUDER THAN WORDS

Look again at some of your own behaviors and the messages that they send:

- ACTION: morning cup of coffee
  MESSAGE: I need a stimulant to get going, give me energy, help me face the day.

- ACTION: a drink after work
  MESSAGE: I need booze to unwind and relax.

- ACTION: drinks on the weekends
  MESSAGE: Alcohol makes football games more fun, conversation easier, parties more enjoyable.

- ACTION: drinks or drugs at parties and get-togethers
  MESSAGE: I need a drink to have fun. Things do go better with "coke."

- ACTION: pills for sleep
  MESSAGE: Pills can make my life run more smoothly.

- ACTION: tranquilizers
  MESSAGE: I need pills to deal with stress.

- ACTION: cigarette with coffee, food, or company
  MESSAGE: I don't enjoy these activities for themselves. I need a crutch even for the little things in life—and drugs are my crutch.

- ACTION: giving an attractive man or woman the eye
  MESSAGE: Physical looks appeal to me more than what's inside the person.

- ACTION: reading sexy magazines or books
  MESSAGE: I often think about having sex with other people.

- ACTION: identifying with characters like seductive James Bond or sultry Marilyn Monroe
  MESSAGE: My goal is sexual conquest.

Of course, if you practice any of these behaviors or others like them, you may have very different reasons for doing so. Yet your reasons are not the point here. It is the message a youngster interprets from your actions that counts. Asking your child to adopt certain behaviors may mean that you may have to change some of your own. Take stock of what your actions say to your child.

"You're too young to be smoking. If I ever catch you sneaking a cigarette at the mall again, you'll be grounded for a good long time!" Martha was livid. She had caught a glimpse of her daughter Jessie smoking in the nearby mall with a group of friends. Jessie was 13 years old, but even if she were 18, Martha wouldn't have wanted her to smoke. "I just don't want you to fall into the same trap I did. I started smoking at your age and I haven't been able to quit since. Smoking is bad for you. For goodness' sake, Jessie, don't follow my bad example."

Jessie mumbled some excuse and an apology, then retreated to her room in tears. Martha began fixing dinner, banging pots and slamming down bottles. She was angry with her family. Jessie was her third child and the third of her children to take up smoking. Martha was angry with herself too. "Telling them to do as I say and not as I do is just not good enough," she told herself. She had tried to quit smoking several times in the past but she had not been successful. With a heavy sigh, she decided to try quitting again. She didn't feel the same energetic confidence she did the times she decided to quit before, but she did feel a heavy burden of responsibility to at least show her daughter that she would try hard to practice what she preached.

As the days grew into weeks, Martha realized that staying away from cigarettes grew easier as Jessie kept encouraging her. She had told Jessie that she was trying to quit in order to show her just how strongly she felt about not wanting her ever to start smoking. Jessie's interest was keen, and she seemed to really understand just how important this was to her mom. It became a battle they fought together: Martha's stopping a 25-year habit, and Jessie trying not to begin one.

Martha had learned that all the words in the world may not give as loud and clear a message as actions. If your expectations for your child and your own actions seem to give a double message, then do something positive for yourself. Change. In doing so you are making a commitment to your child. At the same time, you are making a commitment to yourself by becoming healthier.

"Tell Me You Love Me, Mom and Dad": Parent as Nurturer

Not only do our actions send out messages, but so do the ways in which we relate to our children. In recent years, there has been a shift away from blaming parents for the faults of their children. This has been a healthy shift, removing the heavy burden of guilt from mothers or fathers who may have been less than perfect since the birth of their child. On the other hand, some parents have come to absolve themselves of any responsibility, saying that their child's friends, society at large, or the inner makings he was born with have led to the child's troublesome behaviors.

"We tried so hard. We did everything right to raise her to be good. We can't understand where we went wrong." These well-known words from fiction and from real life can be hypocritical. "We can't understand where we went wrong" is a cliché, but do people who say it really believe that they might have done something out of line? A concerned family should be looking at itself *before* those words become necessary. What can we do better? How are we missing the mark?

Psychological research has shown that not only do parents' behaviors influence the actions of youngsters, so do parents' interactions with their children. Your perceptions of your children do influence how your children perceive themselves.

When you have more than one child, it is easy to begin comparing them. Sarah is quieter and more thoughtful. James is agile and strong. Peter is outgoing. Jenny quietly observes people before talking to them. These comparisons are natural and pretty hard to avoid. By themselves, they probably do no great harm. When the comparisons become labels, however, children may then find themselves trapped in a role they must fulfill.

Take, for example, the classic case of the "black sheep" of the family. Zachary is a good and well-behaved son, but Michael is bad-tempered and always into trouble. Michael has been labeled; everything he does will be interpreted as predictably bad or good-but-what's-the-catch? Once parents have let the labels settle in, the same behavior by Zachary and Michael will trigger different responses from the parents. Zachary's deed will be mischievous and perhaps given a light reprimand. Michael, on the other hand, will just be digging a deeper grave, so to speak, and his punishment will be more severe.

Oddly enough, at other times it is Zachary who suffers. The perfect child will be expected to behave perfectly. His parents expect good grades, popularity, good manners, athletic prowess or whatever is important in their value systems. The stress can be overwhelming. As the expectations become greater, so does the chance for failure. Zachary soon finds himself faced with expectations he can't meet or becomes so afraid of failing that he no longer tries. He drops out from the family network because the strain is too much.

What does your youngster think that you think about her? "She knows we love her," is a typical response. But what does she believe that you think about her as a person? Despite what you imagine, chances are that you don't tell her often enough how proud you are of her or what you admire about her.

"Gee, you really came up with a good solution to that problem. That's pretty smart thinking."

"I'm proud of the way you can stand up for yourself, even when your friends try to get you to do something you don't want to do."

"You have pretty eyes (or hair or face, etc.)."

"I realize we have a difference of opinion about this and I wish you'd see things my way. But I'm glad that you can think things through for yourself."

"You know, I think you've done a pretty good job of living your life."

"I know that the things I ask of you, like not going to un-chaperoned parties, not smoking or drinking, and not dating certain kinds of people, may be asking a lot. It probably is harder to be a young person now than it was when I was young."

"You have done something very wrong. But because you are basically a good kid, I'm going to consider this a one-time mistake that won't happen again."

"I love you. I'm lucky to have you."

Maintaining a positive perspective, however, must be balanced with having a realistic one. Denial, or assuming that everything is A-Okay, is quite common in families. A recent poll showed that 75% of parents reported being certain that their children did not use drugs, but when they were questioned again soon afterwards, the parents expressed more doubt, saying, "These questions made me realize I was assuming too much. I've started to talk to my children more openly since then."

Exercise 16   **PARENT and CHILD**

TELL ME WHO YOU ARE

Every relationship needs renewing. Take time out regularly to look at yourself and your family in order to find out who you are and where you want to go. The following questions are designed for you and your child (or spouse) to ask one another, in confidence and without threat. Complete openness will not come right away, not until you build trust in one another and in these questions. Be willing to take risks, to trust your partner.

You may find that some issues are too touchy to share. If that is the case, respect one another's vulnerability and do not push your partner for an answer. Skip any questions that make either of you feel uncomfortable, for there is always time in the future to learn the answers. And above all, do not use any information against the other person.

This exercise can be used as an interview sheet as you take turns asking each other the same question. You can also write the questions on cards and, after the shuffling the cards, pick one at a time and ask your partner the question on the card. You will find that after a while you will not need these questions—you will have a storehouse of your own, but remember the basic rules of respect.

(continued)

(*Exercise 16 continued*)

What have you always wanted to talk more about?

What would you find fun to do?

In what ways are we the same?

In what ways are we different?

When do we seem to have the most fun together?

When are you proud of me?

When do you feel closest to me?

When do you feel farthest away from me?

How can we be closer?

How can I help you most?

When do you need me most?

What is my greatest strength?

When do I annoy you most?

Have I ever misjudged you?

How do I sometimes hurt you?

What do you think is your greatest strength?

What do you like best about yourself?

What would you like to do in six months, (one, two, more years)?

What do you want me to think of you?

What are your hopes?

What scares you most?

What are the three most important things in the world to you?

Keeping Control Under Control: Parent as Protector

What a difficult line to walk: mistrust hurts, but so does denial. Although it takes a concerted effort, you can trust without wearing blinders and keep tabs on your children without subjecting them to police-style interrogations.

The key is to feel secure in your role as parent, to expect your children to be able to account for their whereabouts and actions when asked. You can temper your inquiries by respecting the rights of your child. Will you make mistakes? Of course. Sometimes you may be faced with an angry adolescent claiming insult. That is okay provided it does not happen too often. At other times you may wish you had kept closer tabs on finding out where your child was going, with whom, for how long, and for what reasons. Again, that is okay, you are not running a police state in your home.

Feeling secure in your role as parent also means feeling comfortable with imposing some controls. The issue of control can be a touchy one—certainly one that can ignite parent-child battles. And again, it can pose a challenge to you to try to maintain that fine line between too little control and too much.

"C'mon Dad, you're treating me like a little kid," Sam's daughter shouted. "All the other kids' parents are letting them go to the 10 o'clock sneak preview of that movie. No one else has to be home by 10:30 on a weekend. You're not letting me grow up." After his daughter fled the room, Sam decided to call one or two of the other parents to see if indeed they were letting their daughters go to such a late show. One call bore out his daughter's testimony. "Well, maybe I am being a little strict," he decided, and then told his daughter that she could join her friends.

Sam was sorry he had changed his mind, however, when his daughter dragged in past 2:00 A.M. She had gone out to get a bite to eat after the show. Asking for special permission and then taking advantage of the situation was not, unfortunately, a new behavior for her. "C'mon Dad, you're treating me like a kid," his daughter once again told him. Sam told his daughter that he had tried to treat her as an older teen, but that she had failed to act responsibly.

"But you didn't tell me when you wanted me home. I can't read your mind. I didn't do anything wrong. I just went to the show and then out to eat," she entreated. She was right. Sam hadn't made clear his expectations. In fact, he had seesawed from being too controlling to not being controlling enough. In talking about everything that happened, Sam admitted that he had been a little too strict in some areas and his daughter agreed that she had tried to push him to his limits.

As a first step, Sam decided to let his daughter stay out an hour later on weekends, but if she was late, he would ground her for the next weekend. Even though his daughter felt she should, like her friends, be able to stay out later than 11:30, she agreed to the new curfew. In return, she asked her Dad to think about extending the curfew another hour if she could prove over the next few months that she could be responsible. Sam thought the idea was reasonable and together they set the curfew and the consequences if the rules were violated.

The goal of both parent and child is to have the child grow into an independent adult. That means the developing child will naturally want more autonomy. At the same time, the parent will need to loosen controls and allow the child to make his own decisions and take responsibility for his actions. The typical tug-of-war between the child who wants more autonomy and the parent who wants to relinquish control more slowly is healthy, often leading to a good compromise position. Your first guide for what is a suitable degree of control can be found somewhere in that area of disagreement between you and your child.

What are some practical tips that can help?

1. As your child grows older, loosen your grip.

2. Slowly scale down to a minimum the number of restrictions and demands you place on your child. The power of the Ten Commandments comes from the fact that there are only ten, not twenty-three or seventy-eight.

3. The fewer the controls, the more they count: your child will know that there are some things you will not accept. Make certain those few controls are for important issues, not trivial ones.

4. Include expectations for yourself as parent. Ask your child to offer some suggestions, such as respecting the privacy of her mail or his wallet.

5. Enforce the controls. Be consistent in your expectations and your reactions; be flexible, however, when uncontrollable circumstances arise to interfere with your child's ability to meet your expectations to the letter. Work out a scheme with your family for making sure expectations are met.

6. Finally, make clear your expectations. Here are suggested guidelines for rules, or expectations, you can share with your family:

   • Curfews must be set and met. Different curfews may apply to weekday and weekend nights.
   • Children must attend school on all school days unless they are ill and have their parents' permission to be absent.
   • Children should tell parents where they are going, why, with whom, and when they will be back home.
   • Children must call their parents if they will be delayed in getting home for any reason.
   • Parents must agree to pick their children up, without reproach, if the youngsters wish to leave a gathering in which alcohol or drugs are being used.
   • Parents and children should know how to reach one another by phone.
   • Parents should know the parents of their children's friends.
   • Parents should be awake to greet children when they come home in the evening.
   • Parties must be chaperoned by an adult.
   • No alcohol or drugs are allowed at parties.
   • Parents must be able to call the party site if necessary.

Working Together Works: Parent as Ally

What brings a country together in response to an outside threat? What brings a city together during the football season? What brings a political faction together during a big election? What can bring a family together?

There is a concept called "superordinate goal." This is a goal that requires more than one person; it can require many people working together to achieve something they all want even though they differ in many other ways. Think back to any projects you may have undertaken for your child. Perhaps you bought your daughter a new bike that came unassembled. If she was old enough to help out, the two of you may have assembled the bike together, both excited about the anticipated finished product. Or perhaps you grew tomato plants with your son, trained a new puppy with your child, cheered for the same sports team.

Now that Mike was in his teens, Sara realized that she and her son found little time to talk to one another. When they did talk, they argued over rules and chores. Sara tried countless times to ask Mike about serious issues such as what he wanted to do when he got older, what kind of influences he was receiving from his friends, and so on. Her attempts were met with silence. About the only time he was really home was during Monday night football games on television.

Sara decided that even if he didn't talk to her, he would have to see her. She wanted him to be aware of her presence if nothing else. So she sat on the chair next to him every Monday evening while he sat with his eyes glued to the television screen. She began to ask him what he was so excited about whenever he jumped up screaming after some football play. Soon Sara began to recognize some of the good plays. She began to develop some allegiances to a couple of the teams and even glanced at the sports page headlines to find out more about them. The more she became interested in the game, the more she and her son talked.

By the end of the season, Sara and her son were having "fun arguments" over who would win the play-off games. Mike hung around the kitchen after school just to talk about sports with his mom. This became a time they counted on and enjoyed. Although the major topic remained sports, both mother and son used the time to talk about other things too. When basketball season came around, Sara and Mike began to cheer for the same team. In fact, the two of them had become quite a team in themselves.

A mutual goal can bring you and your children closer together and open up channels of communication that may have been blocked. Try to find a project or activity that you both care about, that requires some regular involvement. Examples may be:

- Sports—either participatory or spectator—such as bowling, basketball, football, baseball, volleyball, fishing, etc.
- Building projects such as a desk or other furniture for the child's room, a ping-pong table, a dog house.
- Hobbies such as ham radio, model airplanes, stitchery, art.
- Cooking favorite meals or desserts together.
- Camping, hiking, horticulture, or other outdoor activities.
- Helping others: the homeless, the elderly, the mentally retarded, the poor, an invalid neighbor.
- Planning together: vacations, surprises, budgets for a mutually desired item.
- Praying together, giving thanks, taking a moment to enjoy life around you.
- Working together to clean the house, rake the yard, weed the garden, fix the car.
- Learning together.

All these activities can be fun, not drudgery, so try hard to include a sense of enjoyment. Rewards can help too. The reward for building a doghouse may be just the end product itself. The reward for helping cook a meal may be a special dessert treat. The reward for helping clean the yard may be a little extra added to the allowance.

Above all, keep the long-term goal clearly in view. For some things, such as helping the elderly, that is easy and probably does not need many words other than telling your child he is a fine person for helping. For other tasks, such as cleaning house, the goal of having a pleasant, clean-smelling, and welcoming home should be stated.

And be clear about one of your ultimate superordinate goals—raising a happy, healthy child who will grow to be a happy, healthy, independent adult. In working toward this goal—and work it is—stay on your child's side. Do not let your need for control and his need for freedom turn you into adversaries. Work together!

In reality, you cannot truly control anyone, even your child. You can, however, influence those you love. Where does your ultimate control lie? Only within yourself. By trying hard to be the kind of parent you want to be, you are more likely to have a strong influence on your child. Respect your responsibility as a role model. Find little ways as well as big ways to encourage your child and let him know how positive you feel about him. Set limits with confidence and within reason. Work, play, and be with your child.

7

WHAT ARE YOUR VALUES?

We each have our own set of values about what is right or wrong, what is good or bad behavior. For the most part, these values have developed through careful training from parents, teachers, or other adults who were important during our childhood years. Expectations were often made very clear to us: "Don't talk with your mouth full"; "Respect your elders"; "Do unto others"; "Tell the truth"; "Share your toys"; "Clean your plate."

The major roles of parents are to teach their children how to behave and to impart moral values. They often have little difficulty setting standards for their child's behavior in a wide variety of situations, yet when it comes to the areas of sex and drugs, parents often clam up. These are difficult areas to discuss, and rather than risk possible embarrassment or confusion parents often decide to "skip that part."

Although parents often feel uneasy talking about sex, drinking, or drug use with their children, these activities are becoming a part of our children's lives. More and more children are getting involved with these behaviors at earlier ages than ever before. It is difficult for parents to think of their child as a sexual being or as an individual who may find reasons for trying or relying on drugs. One reason for this difficulty may stem from our hesitating to see children as growing up, for we can see so much that is still so childlike about them. Another reason may stem from our having an uncomfortable feeling about such private issues as sex or other deep needs, such as loneliness, that may prompt drug use. Still another reason may be symptomatic of the ostrich syndrome: "If I don't see it, it isn't there."

Some parents rationalize, "My child knows the difference between right and wrong," or, "He'll never get in trouble with drugs or get involved with sex." Is this really true? The statistics on teenage involvement with drugs and sex would not support that statement. Have you clearly explained to your child what behaviors you expect and do not expect of him? Have you really examined your expectations closely? These questions become particularly important when the outcomes of your child's behavior can have such a great impact.

Parents may say that they don't ever want their child to get involved with drugs or sex. These blanket statements do not address the continuum of values that parents may have about the different levels of behavior associated with drugs or sex. For example, some parents may believe it is okay for their child to drink alcohol as long as he does so at home. Others may allow some drinking on special occasions, while still others may forbid any consumption of alcohol.

Similarly, there are a variety of behaviors that can be considered part of sexual contact, and many parents have difficulty determining what is acceptable behavior and what is not. What about holding hands, kissing , fondling? Should a child be taught about birth control? These are all values and expectations that every parent needs to consider. How can a child know what a parent expects if the parent isn't sure?

This book cannot tell you what is right or wrong for your child. You and your child are the only ones who can establish that. What some parents might deem acceptable behavior, others would consider *verboten*. Behaviors that might be prevalent among a group of youngsters in one part of the country might not even exist in another. In establishing the guidelines for what you can expect from your child, you must first define your values, and second, understand your child's values and the norms that exist in your child's circle of friends. Then, let your child know exactly what behaviors you disapprove of, and what the possible consequences of those behaviors might be. But realize that your child may end up experimenting with these "adult" behaviors, and that you will need to decide how to cope with the possibility that your child might make an error of judgment.

When you begin to examine your values, you may become aware that it isn't always easy to find the one "right" answer. There are many issues to consider when thinking about drug use and sexual behavior. You need to explore these issues in depth.

What Are Your Values about Alcohol, Tobacco, and Other Drugs

Legal Drugs

Alcohol and tobacco are legal drugs for persons who are of legal age to use them. Society demonstrates its own set of values when it declares that a person may drink or smoke at a given age. Some parents allow their children to drink alcohol before they are "legal," others do not. Some people allow their children to smoke cigarettes, others forbid them to smoke even though they are of legal age to do so.

We often get our values from what our parents allowed us to do. Some parents might rationalize, "Those seem to be good values because look how well we turned out." The problem with adopting the same values our parents had is that the dynamics are just not the same. You are different from your parents in terms of personality, abilities, needs, and other characteristics. Your children are different from you as a child. The social climate has changed, as have the pressures your children face. Moreover, we have gained more knowledge about drug effects, such as the relationship between cigarette smoking and cancer or the tendency for alcoholism to run in families. Given all these changes from your parents' time, you may still decide to adopt similar values, or you may choose new ones. The point is that you need to actively question your values and not blindly accept those from the past.

Under what circumstances would you allow your child to drink alcohol? Would you allow him to taste it if you were having a drink; have some to celebrate a holiday; drink in the house but not elsewhere? What are your limits and will they change as your child gets older? With the increasing death rates associated with drinking and driving among teenagers, what will you do to try to prevent this from happening to your child?

What about smoking? Many people do not want their children to smoke; some will allow it but only when the child is 16 or 18 or leaves home; some only forbid smoking in the house. What are your values about smoking? Keep in mind that 98% of people who smoke are addicted to tobacco; only 2% can smoke occasionally or quit with no negative side effects. Many smokers are keenly aware of the hazards of smoking and the difficulty in quitting, and they do not want their children to start. It is okay to forbid your child from doing something that you yourself do. It is even better if you can show him your values by your own behavior.

Illegal and Illicit Drugs

Marijuana, cocaine, heroin, LSD, PCP—these are all illegal drugs to the general public. These are also the drugs that parents fear the most, even though their use is much less prevalent than the legal drugs of alcohol and tobacco. Many parents forbid their children to use these drugs; others may allow occasional use or experimentation with marijuana. What are your values and do your children know how you feel?

Some legal drugs or substances become "illicit" when they are used in ways that were not originally intended. Prescription or over-the-counter medications are sometimes abused by teens— pain killers, mood-elevating pills, cough medicines containing alcohol, and other drugs in the medicine cabinet can provide a "high." Similarly, other substances commonly found in the home are frequently abused. Inhaling glue, paint, aerosol sprays, gasoline, or the fluid for correcting typing errors can all produce intoxicating effects. These drugs or substances are available in your home right now. What if your child were using them illicitly to get high?

Experimentation vs. Regular Use

What would you think if your child tried cigarettes, marijuana, or alcohol just once to "see how it feels" with no intention of using it again? The question of experimentation vs. regular use is a big one for parents, because adolescence is a time of increased curiosity and desire to try new things. For many parents, the ability to tolerate experimentation depends on how dangerous the drug is: can it have a lasting effect even if used only once? They believe that permitting a child to experiment, under close supervision and with a "less harmful" drug, helps reduce the mystique of that drug. It no longer becomes the "forbidden fruit" that is all the more desirable because teens are not allowed to have it.

Other parents view experimentation as the first step to regular use and they forbid it entirely. They believe that by allowing a child to experiment with a drug they are actively condoning the use of that drug or the continuing experimentation with forbidden substances.

How do you feel? Examine your values closely and carefully in light of who you are and who you know your child to be.

What Are Your Values about Sexuality?

Parents want their children to grow into adults who can form a strong intimate relationship with someone of the opposite sex, get married, and raise a family. At the core of such relationships is a healthy sexuality.

As you assess your values regarding teen sexuality, avoid defining sexuality as merely the sex act. Sexuality is loving, caring about, and relating to other human beings. A child learns about sexuality at home, from the time he is born and his parents lovingly tend to him. It is a parent's job to help him continue developing a healthy sexuality.

What is an acceptable maturing process for your child? Dating is acceptable in this society as a means for young people to learn how to relate to the opposite sex. What is your stance on dating: age, activities, curfews, whether you meet the date, and so on? Is there a difference between a date at a public social activity and a date in a home while the parents are out?

An important aspect of sexuality is respect for the opposite sex. What pictures have you presented about roles of females or males? Do you hold a different set of standards for girls than for boys? If you do, why? And what message does that send to your children? Many parents cite that the risk of pregnancy is more detrimental to a girl than a boy. But what about the risk of a sexually transmitted disease, especially one that may be incurable, such as herpes or AIDS?

We have left the era of thinking that complete ignorance is bliss, that a boy or girl who does not know about sex will therefore never learn about it nor be tempted by it. Parents do expect that their children will be educated about the biological aspects of sex. But what about contraception—how it works and where to obtain it? Some parents fear that telling their son or daughter about birth control will give implicit approval for engaging in sex. Studies of sex education programs, however, have shown that there is no increase in sexual activity among students who have learned about contraception. Other parents tell their children "I don't approve of your engaging in sex and don't think you will; however, I feel you should learn about contraception because I don't want an unwanted pregnancy to arise from any mistakes you might make."

If you do not want to tell your child about contraception, how will you deal with the (mis)information she gets from peers? What if your child does become sexually active but has not learned how to use, or has not used, protection? How will you deal with the possible consequences: abortion, adoption, or trying to make the new teenage family work? What are your expectations if your son fathers a baby? If you do want your child to know about contraception, who will tell him or her? Will you? Do you want someone else to, such as teachers, youth organizers or health care providers? And when should your child learn?

What about "safe sex" techniques? If you think your child may already be sexually active, are you sure he or she knows how to protect against sexually transmitted diseases, including AIDS? How will you deal with this issue?

Your values about sex and about how your child should express his or her sexuality are difficult issues to face, and the questions posed in this section may cause some discomfort. Yet the issues are real. And the issues are ones that your child will actively think about in formulating his own values.

Defining Your Values

In the activity entitled "Clarifying Your Expectations," there is one exercise pertaining to drug and alcohol use (Exercise 17) and one that discusses sexual behavior (Exercise 18). These exercises are designed to promote an awareness of your own values about what is right and wrong for your child. Before you say "My child knows what I expect," check to make sure that *you* know what you expect. Once you have completed the exercises, save your answers. They will be useful in later chapters when you and your child begin to establish your own ground rules for acceptable behavior.

Bear in mind that values change. Sometimes they change as your child matures. For example, hand-holding may be the extent of allowable physical intimacy for a 13-year-old, but kissing may be allowable, and certainly normal, for a 16-year-old. Similarly, a sip of champagne at big brother's wedding may be permissible for a 14-year-old, while a cold beer may in some households cap off a hard weekend of summertime chores for a 20-year-old.

Values can also change because consequences change. For example, the threat of herpes and AIDS has influenced the values about sexuality—for both teens and adults. Likewise, as the health effects of smokeless tobacco and nontobacco cigarettes become better known, individuals may find these less acceptable alternatives to cigarette use.

Your values may also undergo change as circumstances become different. For example, you may believe that your child should not have sexual intercourse before marriage. If you find that he or she has become sexually active, the focus of your concern might shift from maintaining virginity to preventing pregnancy or protecting against disease.

It is therefore important to reassess your values over time. As your values change, for one reason or another, let your children know. Remember, too, that young people change their values—that's a part of growing up. Keep in touch; find out how your child's values develop.

Considering the Bottom Line

Even more difficult to consider is that there are issues about

Exercise 17 **PARENT**

CLARIFYING YOUR EXPECTATIONS ABOUT DRUGS

Listed below are various drugs and levels of drug use. In the left-hand column, write the age at which you would tolerate your child engaging in each level. In the right-hand column, write the age at which your child may actually engage in the behavior, with or without your approval. Write NEVER if you believe your child would never participate in a behavior or if you would never tolerate it.

	MY CHILD'S AGE WHEN PARTICIPATING	
	What I could Accept	What Could Happen

Tobacco

Try a few puffs	_____	_____
Smoke a whole cigarette	_____	_____
Smoke a few times a year	_____	_____
Smoke a few times a month	_____	_____
Smoke a few times a week	_____	_____
Smoke a few cigarettes a day	_____	_____
Smoke half a pack a day	_____	_____
Smoke a pack or more a day	_____	_____

Alcohol

Try a sip of beer or wine	_____	_____
Try a sip of liquor	_____	_____
Have a whole drink at home	_____	_____
Have a whole drink with friends	_____	_____

(continued)

(Exercise 17 continued)

Drink a few times a year _____ _____
Drink a few times a month _____ _____
Drink a few times a week _____ _____
Drink daily _____ _____

Marijuana

Try a puff _____ _____
Share a whole joint with friends _____ _____
Smoke a few times a year _____ _____
Smoke a few times a month _____ _____
Smoke once a week _____ _____
Smoke once a day _____ _____

Other Drug (_____)

Experiment once _____ _____
Use once a year or less _____ _____
Use once a month _____ _____
Use a few times a month _____ _____
Use once a week _____ _____
Use a few times a week _____ _____
Use daily _____ _____

What are the reasons you have for the limits you have set for:

Tobacco use _____

_____

Alcohol use _____

_____

Marijuana use _____

_____

Other drug use _____
(_____) _____

_____

Exercise 18   **PARENT**

CLARIFYING YOUR EXPECTATIONS
ABOUT SEXUALITY

Listed below are levels of sexual behavior. In the left-hand column, write the age at which you would tolerate your child engaging in each level. In the right-hand column, write the age at which your child may actually engage in the behavior, with or without your approval. Write NEVER if you believe your child would never participate in a behavior or if you would never tolerate it.

	MY CHILD'S AGE WHEN PARTICIPATING	
	What I Could Accept	What Could Happen
Talking on the phone	_____	_____
Going on a date	_____	_____
Holding hands	_____	_____
Kissing briefly	_____	_____
Prolonged kissing	_____	_____
Hugging or holding	_____	_____
Caressing the body over clothing	_____	_____
Caressing the body under clothing	_____	_____
Fondling to orgasm	_____	_____
Sexual intercourse	_____	_____
Other:		
_____	_____	_____
_____	_____	_____

(continued)

(Exercise 18 continued)

Now answer the following questions:

1. Do you believe it is your duty to tell your child about sex? (If not, who should?) When should your child become informed? _____

_____

2. Do you believe it is your duty to tell your child about birth control or "safe sex" techniques? (If not, who should?) When should your child become informed? _____

_____

3. If you learned that your child was sexually active, how would you react? _____

_____

4. If your daughter became pregnant or your son was responsible for a pregnancy, what would you do?

_____

_____

5. On a scale of 1 to 10—extremely easy to extremely difficult—how difficult was it for you to think about or answer the questions in this exercise? Why?_____

_____
_____
_____
_____

which children hold different values than their parents. Regardless of what parents expect from their children, there may be times when even the best of kids does something against his parents' wishes. For example, parents may be extremely opposed to teenage drinking or sexual activity, but the statistics indicate that many teens will engage in these behaviors regardless of their parents' views. What should you do?

Let's take the example of drinking. An organization called Students Against Drunk Driving, or S.A.D.D., has developed a contract that parents and their children can sign. It simply states that if the child has been drinking or is with a driver who has been drinking, then the child agrees to call the parents for a ride home; no questions asked until later.

Does this mean that the parents *condone* their child's drinking? Not in the least. It means that the parents recognize the possibility that their child might drink, and although they disapprove of it, the "bottom line" is that they do not want him to get hurt in a car accident.

The same rules may apply to teenage sexuality. Many parents fear that by telling their child about birth control, they are encouraging sexual activity. This is not true. In fact, it may help teenagers realize the serious consequences of having sex if they are forced to consider the reality of an unwanted pregnancy. If you disapprove, let your child know, but don't stop there. Your child may choose to be sexually active anyway, and the bottom line is that an unwanted pregnancy should be avoided. Teaching your child about "safe sex" practices to avoid a serious sexually transmitted disease can at one level illustrate that sex cannot be a casual pleasure while at another level safeguarding your child's health and possibly his life from unrestrained submission to temptation.

Is it more important that your child not drink or that he not get killed in a car accident while driving drunk? Granted, if he didn't do the former, the latter wouldn't happen, but can you count on the fact that he will never drink? Let him know that even if he has the bad judgment to drink, you would rather he call you for help than try to hide it from you and risk getting killed. Or if your daughter goes against your rules and decides to have sex, let her know where she can get information about birth control so that her bad decision does not result in an unwanted pregnancy.

Now go back to the exercises you completed on "Clarifying Your Expectations." As you review the column on what could happen, consider your "bottom line" values. What can you do now to prevent any mistakes your child might make from becoming a tragedy?

If you and your child share a good relationship based on trust and mutual responsibility, chances are the choices he makes for himself will be the same as the ones you would make for him. Most youngsters don't want to get involved with drugs; many are hesitant about becoming sexually active. A study of pregnant teenage girls indicated that most didn't intend to get pregnant, or even to have intercourse. "It just happened," they told researchers. This discrepancy between values and action is particularly sad because it could be avoided.

Prepare your children to avoid the "it just happened" syndrome. Teach them to assert themselves, to weigh consequences in order to strengthen their resolve, to say NO when it really counts, to recognize when they need help and to know where to turn.

Instill a sense of confidence and good judgment by rewarding your child for positive behaviors. Set the pattern now for letting her know what she is doing *right*. Chances are that there will be fewer *wrong* behaviors, not only now but in the future as well.

8

THINK POSITIVE

The preceding chapter focused on your values and beliefs about drugs and sex, and on how you think your child "should" behave. Let's step back for a moment and take a look at behaviors in general—how they develop, how they can be changed, and how aware we are of what our children are really doing.

All too often we focus on what is wrong, what needs to be changed, what needs to be avoided. "He didn't come home on time." "She always interrupts." "He didn't finish all of his homework." "She looks overweight." "He forgot to take out the garbage."

Sometimes parents do this as a way of providing guidance in the face of both their own and their child's uncertainty about what lies ahead in the coming years.

"Don't go out without finishing your homework."
"I *don't* like the friends you hang around with."
"Don't you ever let me catch you drinking or you'll wish you hadn't."
"How many times have I told you *not* to throw your clothes on the floor?"

Parents sometimes feel an obligation to tell their children what *not* to do, or to punish them when they do the *wrong* thing, because that's what parents are "supposed" to do. All too often they neglect to focus on exactly what they want their child *to* do and fail to reward her when she does the *right* thing.

Punishments vs. Rewards

When we punish children for doing something wrong, there is a good chance that they will not do it again or will do it less often. Punishment is effective because it stops a behavior, produces quick results, and is usually remembered by the child. Punishment is sometimes necessary, particularly in serious or dangerous situations, because you need to make your point fast. But punishment has several drawbacks:

- It makes both the child and the parent feel angry or resentful.
- Your child may associate punishment with you rather than with the wrong behavior, and either avoid you or do the behavior when you are not around.
- Your child learns that the most effective way of changing others' behaviors is by punishing them.
- Your child doesn't learn how to decide what is right or wrong; he simply learns to react to external controls (punishment).
- The effects of punishment don't last too long; they wear off.
- Your child learns what *not* to do, but does not learn what *to* do.

Giving a child a reward for doing something right increases the probability that he will do it again. Unlike punishment, rewards make the child feel good about himself and his parents, strengthening their relationship. The child learns to appreciate the value of a "right" behavior because it is associated with good things. The effects of rewarding a desired behavior generally last longer than the effects of punishing an undesirable behavior.

It is harder to give children rewards for good behavior because it means that you have to be alert to *all* behaviors. It is easy to notice bad behavior, but when was the last time you noticed good behavior? Rewarding good behavior also means that you must tell your child exactly what you *expect* her to do, and you must consistently reinforce that behavior.

Parents often argue, "He *knows* what I expect him to do without my having to spell it out," or "She should do the right thing without having to be rewarded or 'bribed'." Let's look at each of these arguments.

He knows what I expect. Is this really true? Have you clearly explained to your child what behaviors you expect him to do and not do? Have you really examined your expectations closely? If you completed the exercises in chapter 7, you may have found that even on topics that are crucial to your child's development, such as drugs and sex, your expectations were not completely clear to you. If they are not clear to you, imagine what a difficult time your child will have guessing what your expectations are about his sexual behavior or his future use of alcohol or drugs.

She should do it without having to be rewarded. Granted, we should not have to "buy" proper behavior all the time, but, then again, we should not expect it to occur all the time if it is not reinforced. Would you continue to work if your boss decided to stop paying you a salary because "It's everyone's duty to contribute to society"? Or if you spent hours preparing a fancy meal and no one acknowledged your efforts, would you be eager to do so again? The point is to instill in your child the kinds of behaviors that connote maturity of judgment, compassion for others, and responsibility. And sometimes the price to pay for achieving these behaviors may be an occasional reward.

What Are Your Expectations?

Using Exercise 19, make a list of some expectations you have about your child's behaviors. What do you expect him to do or not do? Think about behaviors that fall into the different realms of your child's world. For example, what expectations might you have about his behaviors at home, at school, in social situations, in interactions with siblings, or in any other situations? Be sure to include some behaviors that your child already does that meet your expectations.

When making the list, try to be as specific as possible about what you would like to see. It helps to imagine that you are describing the behavior to an alien from another planet. The more

Exercise 19   **PARENT**

WHAT ARE YOUR EXPECTATIONS?

Fill in the space below each heading with two or three answers. Be specific in describing behaviors.

At home, I expect my child to:

1. _____
2. _____
3. _____

At school, I expect my child to:

1. _____
2. _____
3. _____

When we are out in public together, I expect my child to:

1. _____
2. _____
3. _____

When going out with his/her friends, I expect my child to:

1. _____
2. _____
3. _____

With brother(s) or sister(s), I expect my child to:

1. _____
2. _____
3. _____

Other behaviors I expect from my child are:

1. _____
2. _____
3. _____

specific you are about your expectations, the less chance there is for misinterpretations. For example, instead of noting that you expect your child to "do his best in school," you might specify that you want him to "complete his homework assignments each night" or "arrive on time to class."

Once you have made the list, review it. Are your expectations reasonable? This is often hard to determine, and you may want to seek the opinion of someone whose judgment you trust, such as your spouse, a neighbor or friend who has children, or another adult. Once you feel comfortable that your expectations are reasonable, check them out with your child. Does she agree with them? Why or why not? Listen carefully to her reasons—the more opposed your child is to a particular expectation, the less likely she will be to adopt the behavior you expect.

What's in it for Your Child?

What sort of things motivate your child? Psychologists call these "reinforcers," because they strengthen a behavior or increase the probability that a behavior will occur. For example, your child will more likely clean her room if her allowance depends upon it than if there is no such contingency. Similarly, your child will spend more time studying if you praise her for her efforts than if you give no recognition.

Each person has different interests, different motivators, different values. It is important to find out just what reinforcers are effective with *your* child. How do you find that out? *Ask your child directly.* You may have noticed that this advice has been a repeated theme throughout the book. That is because a direct line of communication is the most powerful and most efficient way of finding out what you want to know. A lack of communication is probably the biggest problem faced by the majority of families.

You may assume you know what is reinforcing to your child, but you may not always be correct. Granted, if your child has been begging you for weeks to let him go to some event, you can assume that the privilege of going would be a strong reinforcer. However, don't assume that what is reinforcing to you is also reinforcing to your child. Consider the following example:

A mother was trying to get her teenage son to improve his posture and stand up straighter. She would praise him whenever she saw him standing tall. Much to her chagrin, this seemed to make him slouch almost immediately. When questioned, her son told her that the praise was not something appreciated. In fact, it made him embarrassed whenever she did it in front of his friends. What he did want from her was permission to use the family car. When sitting up straight earned minutes behind the wheel of the car, her son's posture began to look like that of a Marine at attention.

Not everyone would be willing to let their child earn driving privileges. Just as reinforcers differ for each child, the kinds of reinforcers a parent is willing to give will be different for each parent. When you and your child make your list of reinforcers in Exercise 20, be honest about what you are willing to use as a reinforcer. Don't promise something you can't or won't deliver. Have in mind some alternatives that you think your child might like.

Don't forget about existing reinforcers when you are making your list. If your child already gets an allowance, you should list that as a reinforcer. If your child has the privilege of going out on weekends or staying out until a certain time, list those things too. Just as the last section asked you to list expectations your child already meets, this section asks you to list reinforcers your child already receives.

Monetary reinforcers, such as material goods or actual payment, can be effective, but don't limit yourself to these. Parents may come to resent the costs of rewarding their child if the rewards are entirely monetary. Moreover, a strictly monetary reward system sends a strong message to your child about the overvaluation of money. Be imaginative in creating reinforcers.

Consider these options: Are there certain people with whom your child would like to spend time? What special places would your child like to visit? Is there a privilege your child would particularly like to earn? Are there things your child would like to hear you say to him that make him feel good? Can you give your child special time or certain favors that make her feel good? Are there special foods or treats he would like to receive? What kinds of activities does your child enjoy?

Set a time with your child to make a list of reinforcers using the categories provided in Exercise 20 or adding new ones.

The Other Side of the Coin

Working for reinforcers and being rewarded for accomplishing new goals is very much a part of life, and parents who reinforce the behaviors they expect from their child are likely to see more positive behaviors. On the other hand, it is equally important for your child to learn that engaging in behaviors that you forbid is going to cost her something she covets, such as one of her reinforcers. Psychologists call this a "response cost," or the price one has to pay for choosing unacceptable behaviors.

Response costs need to be specified as clearly as expectations and reinforcers. They may often simply be the opposite of the reinforcer. For example, your daughter may earn the privilege of spending the night with a girlfriend if she cleans her room. If she chooses not to clean her room, the response cost for that decision is that she cannot spend the night with her friend. On the other hand, response costs can entail actually taking something away. For example, your son has been playing on the baseball team at school. You may set the stipulation that if he does not maintain a "C" average on his report card, he will lose the privilege of playing with the team.

Response costs may involve the loss of existing privileges, the loss of the opportunity to earn rewards, the loss of activities, or even the loss of possessions earned. As much as possible, however, it is recommended that parents focus more on reinforcing positive behaviors rather than taking things away for negative behaviors. If a particular behavior is very important and/or very hard to change, parents may want to use both reinforcers and response costs. The use of response costs will be demonstrated in examples on the following pages.

Setting up a Contract

Now that you have your list of expected behaviors and your list of reinforcers, you and your child are ready to set up a contract.

Exercise 20   **PARENT and CHILD**

WHAT'S IN IT FOR YOUR CHILD?

Together with your child, write down a list of items your child really likes under each category. These can be things s/he already has or does, or things s/he would like to earn.

People I Like To Be With   **Places I Like To Go**

_____   _____
_____   _____
_____   _____
_____   _____

Privileges I Value   **Material Things I Like**

_____   _____
_____   _____
_____   _____

Special Foods I Like   **Activities I Enjoy**

_____   _____
_____   _____
_____   _____
_____   _____

Other Rewards or Favors

_____
_____
_____
_____

This list can provide you with reinforcers or rewards for desired behaviors. Have your child circle the most important items on this list. These will be the most powerful reinforcers.

The purpose of a contract is to document your negotiations clearly so that both sides are aware of exactly what is expected of each person. That way there will be no disagreements about whether or not the expectations have been met or the reinforcers delivered as originally intended. It's all there in black and white.

You and your child must both sign the contract, so it is critical that you both agree on the contingencies. If your child thinks you expect too drastic a behavior change, she probably won't agree to it and it won't happen. On the other hand, if you believe the reinforcer is much too extravagant, you probably won't agree to deliver it. This is where negotiations come into the picture. The art of successful negotiation demands open communication and a willingness to reach a solution in which both parties can benefit.

Encourage your child to become active in setting up goals or devising reinforcers. You might ask such questions as "Do you think that accomplishing this goal will be too difficult in the first week?", or "That reinforcer is a bit too big for this goal. Can you think of something that might be fairer?" The more your child participates in the negotiations, the better chance he will adhere to the contract.

Setting up a contract allows your child to take responsibility for his actions in a mature way. You no longer have to play the "bad guy," constantly reminding him of his responsibilities. It is up to him to fulfill his contract. Parents are often gratified by the freedom they feel in not having to constantly monitor their child to see if she has "done the dishes" or "started her homework." Once a child realizes that it's her responsibility to fulfill the contract without being reminded, she will quickly take the initiative to do so if the reinforcer is important enough to her.

With these ideas in mind, let's set up an example of a contract. In the beginning stages, make your contracts simple with only a few behavioral goals and reinforcers. Once you become more familiar with the process you can become more elaborate. Follow these steps:

1. Decide on two behavioral goals: one your child already does well and one that you and he agree needs improvement.

2. Clearly describe these goals, being sure to specify how often or how long the behavior should occur or any criteria you might have for how well your child must do.
3. Spell out the reinforcers your child will earn for completing the behaviors. If there are response costs in your contract, specify what the cost of not meeting the behavioral goal will be.
4. Sign and date the contract and set up a date to review it.

Example

Susan, a 12-year-old, brought home a note from her teacher. In the note, the teacher indicated that Susan's homework was often late or incomplete, and that as a result Susan's grades were falling. Susan's parents were very concerned. In reviewing the situation, they realized that Susan had been spending most of her evenings watching television, then quickly completing her homework just before bedtime. They decided to make a contract with her.

They talked to Susan about privileges she might want to earn as a result of working on this new behavior, and she said that she would like to spend more time practicing soccer with her father on Saturdays. They also identified another school-related behavior that Susan was already able to do well—arriving on time to class and returning home on time. Susan's parents decided to reinforce this responsible behavior by allowing her the privilege of spending the night with a friend or inviting a friend over every two weeks, as long as she continued to be on time each day.

Their contract looked like this:

Behavior: Complete homework before watching TV without having to be reminded

Reinforcer: One hour with Dad on Saturday to practice soccer

Behavior: Arrive on time to school each day and be home 20 minutes after school ends

Reinforcer:	Permission to spend the night with a friend or invite a friend over for the night every two weeks
Signatures:	_____
	_____
Review date:	every Saturday morning

Reviewing the contract allows both parent and child to assess any changes in behavior and decide on how effective their agreement has been. Maybe Susan's homework habits haven't changed in two weeks, and her parents feel a need to add on a "response cost," such as "no TV during the week until your teacher says your performance is better." Maybe Susan has been doing her homework well, but she is no longer interested in soccer and wants to set up another reinforcer. Or maybe the homework is no longer an issue and other behaviors have become more important to target. If modifications are made on the contract, both parent and child must agree to them.

Example

As another example, let's look at Charlie, a 16-year-old who has just gotten his driver's license. Charlie would love to take the family car out by himself, but his parents are worried that he won't use good judgment and will go places they've forbidden him to go. Many times, parents and children find themselves in a "Catch 22" situation.

Parent: You can't do that because you're not responsible.
Child: I can't prove I'm responsible because you won't give me a chance to show you.

Setting a contract can be a first step in negotiating that responsibility.

Charlie would like to take the car out on a weeknight with his friends. Charlie's parents are not quite ready to let him have

110

the car at night until he demonstrates that he can (a) drive well in the dark, and (b) be reliable in bringing the car back on time He agrees to drive after dark with Dad until Dad feels Charlie has good night-driving skills. In addition, he negotiates with his parents to take the car out only during the day, with the understanding that if he comes home on time on ten consecutive occasions, they will allow him to take the car out one evening a week.

Behavior(s):
- Drive with Dad after dark to establish night-driving skills. Dad will decide, based on performance, when Charlie is capable of driving at night.
- Drive only during the day with permission.
- Have the car home promptly 10 times in a row.

Reinforcement: If Charlie follows the rules, he can take the car out one evening a week to drive someplace approved of by parents.

Response Cost: If Charlie fails to have the car home on time, goes any place he's not supposed to go, or drives carelessly, all driving privileges will be suspended and must be renegotiated.

Signatures: _____

_____

Review Date: 2 weeks

Charlie's desire to drive, and his realization that he needed to earn that privilege, motivated him to be more aware of his responsibilities with the car. By sticking to the rules he also earned his parents' trust.

Reviewing the Contract

It is extremely important to review the contract on a regular basis for a number of reasons. First, it is important to give reinforcers immediately after they have been earned to strengthen the new behavior. Changing a behavior is very difficult to do, and immediate rewards increase the likelihood that the new behavior will be repeated. Frequent reviews of the contract help parents and children become aware of the progress being made.

Second, some contracts may seem perfect at first, yet flaws may become evident later. Reviewing the contract gives both parties a chance to renegotiate if things are not working out as planned. Finally, when reviewing the contract, parents have the opportunity to provide encouragement and praise to their children. With time, the sense of accomplishment and pride a child feels after reaching a goal may become more important than the reinforcers he receives.

Advantages of Making Contracts

1. Expectations are clear, so children know exactly what they are supposed to do.
2. Rewarding a child for good behavior increases his sense of self-esteem and improves the quality of parent-child relationships.
3. The child assumes responsibility for her actions, which leads to more maturity in making decisions.
4. Parents do not have to remind their child constantly about what to do.
5. There is less feeling of guilt about withholding privileges if the child has an opportunity to earn them but chooses not to do so.
6. Parents are likely to see more positive behaviors in a child who is rewarded and praised.

The very act of making a contract means that parents are giving up some control over their child's behavior and placing the responsibility on her to act appropriately. Although many parents find it difficult to relinquish that control, there are many advantages to doing so. First, maintaining total control takes too much energy and is not really possible.

Second, if you are in total control, then who is to blame when your child misbehaves? You! That can lead to a lot of resentment and guilt on your part. Why should *you* be held accountable for every action of your child? Finally, promoting self-control in your child makes him more responsible for his own behaviors. Self-control and independence are goals that parents must encourage if they want their children to become mature, responsible adults. Let your child practice taking responsibility for himself by making a contract with you.

Make a Contract about Drugs or Sex

Contracts can be made to change behaviors, but they can also be made to *prevent* behaviors from starting. In chapter 7 you outlined your expectations about your child's level of drug use and sexual behavior. Let your child know what you expect, what he will earn by complying, and what consequences will follow if he chooses not to comply. The following examples show how this might be done.

Tracy

Tracy's grandfather died of lung cancer, and her father was vehemently opposed to smoking. He knew that many of her friends were experimenting with cigarettes, and he didn't want Tracy to get started. He decided to make a contract with Tracy and reward her for each year she stayed away from cigarettes. They sat down and talked about her grandfather and about peer pressure to try cigarettes. Tracy's father told her that he would give her $100 on January 1st of each year as long as she didn't smoke. He agreed to accept her word if she said she hadn't smoked. If he found out she had smoked without telling him, however, it would cost her $100 . . . and her father's trust.

Tracy and her father also discussed the other consequences of starting smoking: it would cost money, it might injure her health, her clothes would smell, her teeth would look yellow, and some people would not want to be around her when she smoked. On the other hand, smoking would allow her to remain friends with peers who smoke, and she felt smoking made her look mature. For Tracy, the rewards for not smoking clearly outweighed any advantages of smoking, making it much easier to resist the temptation to experiment with her friends.

Jimmy

Jimmy was entering a new high school in an area where drugs were popular among teenagers. His parents let him know that they expected him to stay away from drugs. They told him that they would allow him to go out on weekends and let him use the car as long as no drugs were involved. Jimmy was a good student and wanted to go to college, and his parents agreed to help him with tuition as long as he remained drug-free throughout high school. They put this agreement in a contract.

Also in the contract were specific consequences Jimmy would face if he decided to use drugs. His parents told him they would suspend his driving privileges, restrict his social activities, notify his school counselor and his friends' parents, and seek psychological help if necessary. Jimmy's parents made the costs of using drugs very unpleasant, and the rewards for not using them very appealing.

As the examples suggest, parents can influence their children's choices about drug use and sexual behavior in a positive way that helps promote a healthy self-esteem. If you and your child share a good relationship based on trust and mutual responsibility, chances are the choices he makes for himself will be the same as the ones you would make for him. Use the form at the end of this chapter for establishing a contract with your child about drug use, sexual behavior, or other behaviors you want to work on.

By rewarding your child for positive behaviors, you help instill a sense of confidence and good judgment. Set the pattern now for letting her know what she is doing *right*. Chances are that there will be fewer *wrong* behaviors, not only now but in the future as well.

CONTRACT

Starting Date: _____

Behavior: _____
_____
_____

Reinforcer: _____
_____
_____

Behavior: _____
_____

Reinforcer: _____
_____
_____

Any Response Costs?: _____
_____
_____

Signatures: _____
_____

Review Date: _____

9

FINDING ALTERNATIVES

Human beings have an instinctive drive to fulfill certain basic needs for food, shelter, and sex. We are motivated to seek pleasure and avoid pain. These factors are part of our biological make-up; they are what allow us to survive. While these basic drives promote survival, they can become exaggerated.

Throughout history, humans have been ingesting drugs to experience altered states of consciousness that are pleasurable. The search for the perfect "high" is not unique to our culture or our times. Historical accounts of drug use date back thousands of years, as do accounts of punitive measures that society has used to place limits on drug use.

Similarly, sexual activity has obviously been going on since the beginning of mankind. We can assume that not all sexual activity was prompted solely by biological needs to reproduce the species. Let's face it, human beings have learned that taking drugs or having sex makes them feel good, and this knowledge has been with us a long time. It is no wonder then that adolescents are intrigued by these pleasurable behaviors. The additional lure of sex and drug use for adolescents is that these behaviors are "adult," and may be "forbidden" to them. These temptations come at a time when adolescents so desperately want to *be* adults.

Adolescents, like other human beings, have needs: to feel important, to feel loved, to experience physical pleasure, to feel satisfied, to get excited, to be an individual. These and other needs often lead them to try drugs, sex, or other risk-taking behaviors. Parents might wish that their children would just "sit

116

on those needs" until they become adults, when they can make more "responsible" decisions about how to meet those needs. We cannot expect children to deny the needs that they have, nor is it healthy for them always to do so. Using drugs or sex to fulfill these needs is not, however, the answer; the risks involved most certainly outweigh the momentary gains.

Simply telling teens about the risks of drug use or sexual intercourse will not deter them from engaging in those behaviors—most teens are sure that "it won't happen to me." Information alone is not enough; it does not fulfill the needs that motivate such behaviors. The problem, therefore, is to find *alternative* ways to meet these needs.

Motivators

People are motivated to use drugs or to get involved in sex for different reasons. They are also motivated *not* to engage in these behaviors for other reasons. By looking at both sets of motivators, we can find alternative ways of maximizing pleasure and minimizing risk.

Because the things that motivate each person are different, it is important to take a look at what is most important to *your child*. If an adolescent feels lonely and unloved, she may be motivated to become intimately involved with a boyfriend to ease those feelings. Another adolescent may be motivated to do the same thing not out of loneliness, but out of curiosity or excitement. Similarly, one teen may be motivated to resist sexual activity out of fear of contracting a sexually transmitted disease, while another's motivation to resist may be fear of getting a bad reputation among her friends. Each child is a unique individual, with different motivations, needs, and desires.

Mark, a 15-year-old, had recently started hanging around with a gang of guys who were a few years older than him. Many of the guys smoked cigarettes, and it was rumored that they drank beer and raced their cars along the side streets. Mark's parents were worried about his choice of friends, and told him they did not approve of them. They asked him what made those guys so much fun to be around. Mark said, "I can't even drive yet. Hanging around them makes me feel older. Riding around with them may be kind of dangerous at times, but it's exciting! They really know how to have fun."

Mark admitted that some of his other friends didn't respect him when he hung around with the gang. While he didn't like their bad reputation, he sure liked the fun the gang had. Mark's father thought of an alternative way to get that same excitement without the bad reputation and he presented it to Mark.

There was a group of guys and their fathers who liked racing dirt bikes (motorcycles) on a track outside of town. The group had strict safety guidelines about racing, but they had a lot of fun and even entered competitions throughout the county. Mark and his father started getting involved with the dirt bike group and soon Mark was no longer interested in the other gang.

Find out what motivates your son or daughter. In Exercise 21, you and your child will make a list of the kinds of things that motivate adolescents' decisions about drug use and sexual behavior. Approach this exercise with an open mind and an attitude of trying to understand. Your acknowledgement of the pleasurable aspects of drugs or sex does not mean you condone such behaviors for teens—it simply means you want to understand them. Use this opportunity to solicit your child's opinion of why teens do *not* engage in these behaviors. Provide reasons of your own that your child may not have considered.(Note: These will become important in the next chapter when your child will be considering consequences of drug use and sex in making decisions.)

Be sure to spend time thinking of as many motivators as you can. Continually ask your child, "Can you think of another reason why kids use drugs?" or "What other things motivate kids to avoid sex?" If you get stuck, there is a list of motivators that have been elicited from groups of adolescents on page 122. Refer to this list only after you have exhausted your combined efforts.

Your child may feel defensive or uncomfortable while complet-

118

Exercise 21   **PARENT**

WHY DO THEY DO WHAT THEY DO?
A Parent's Opinions

Parents are to write their answers on this page. The next page is for the child's answers.

Under each question, list as many reasons as you can think of to answer that question.

Parent's List   **Child's List** (fill in later)

Some teens in your child's school drink or take drugs. Why?

_____   _____
_____   _____
_____   _____

Some teens do not drink or take drugs. Why not?

_____   _____
_____   _____
_____   _____

Some teens in your child's school are sexually active. Why?

_____   _____
_____   _____
_____   _____

Some teens are not sexually active. Why not?

_____   _____
_____   _____
_____   _____

When you both have finished, have your child write his or her answers in the column next to yours. Discuss your answers and add more if you think of them later.

Then ask your child to circle one reason under each heading that seems to be the most important motivator for that behavior.

Exercise 21   **CHILD**

WHY DO THEY DO WHAT THEY DO?
A Teen's Opinions

Teens are to write their answers on this page.

Under each question, list as many reasons as you can think of to answer that question.

Some teens in school drink or take drugs. Why?

_____

_____

_____

Some teens in your school do not drink or take drugs. Why not?

_____

_____

_____

Some teens in your school are sexually active. Why?

_____

_____

_____

Some teens in your school are not sexually active. Why not?

_____

_____

_____

When you have finished, share your answers with your parent and compare the answers you both gave. Then follow the directions at the bottom of your parent's answer sheet.

ing the exercise. If so, you may need to become more spontaneous in presenting the ideas in the exercise. Has there been a recent TV show or newspaper article about teenage drug use or sexuality? Use that show or article as a topic of discussion, and ask your child to give you his or her opinion about why teenagers get involved with drugs or sex.

Examining the Motivators

This chapter focuses mainly on the reasons why teenagers are attracted to drugs and sex. By examining these motivators, parents and their children can begin to explore alternative activities that can be equally attractive without the negative effects that can often accompany drug use or sexual behavior. Before we look more closely at motivators to engage in those behaviors, let's examine some of the reasons that teenagers list for *not* getting involved. These may be helpful for those people who had difficulty listing such reasons in the previous exercise.

Reasons for not *taking drugs:* get addicted; costs money; ruin your health; bad reputation; get caught; act dumb when "high"; smell bad; ruin your appearance; disappoint family; don't need it to feel good; against religious beliefs

Reasons for not *being sexually active:* possible pregnancy; bad reputation; get herpes; get AIDS; disappoint parents; against religious beliefs; keep virginity until married; get caught; wait until meet the right person

Now let's focus on the things that attract teenagers to those behaviors. The reasons your child circled as being the most important motivators for drug use and sexuality may reflect his own values and possibly those of his peer group. Although you can't always assume that these reasons are the most influential ones, look at them and see if you can determine a pattern for your child. Usually the motivators fall into one or more of six categories. These categories are listed on page 122, along with examples of each.

Social Acceptance
fit in with the crowd; afraid to be different; want to look cool; others doing it; friend wants to share; expected by peers; popular people do it; part of social norms; feel close to someone; want to be loved or be in love

Pleasure Seeking
have a good time; do something exciting; makes you feel good; makes pleasurable activities even more fun; thrilling; get "high"; feel satisfied

Self-Esteem Enhancement
look or feel more mature; feel independent; feel sexually attractive; feel lovable; less critical of self; feel okay and competent; gain others' approval

Escape
forget about problems; get into yourself; avoid thoughts of hurtful events; don't have to think about responsibilities; escape from depression; anesthetize self from bad feelings

Stress Reduction
physically relax and unwind; get rid of boredom; let mind wander; release of sexual tension; less nervous under pressure

Risk Taking
curiosity; rebel against authority; try something dangerous; take a chance; thrill of almost getting caught; excitement of getting away with it; prove you're not afraid

Alternatives

There are numerous ways to meet the needs that drugs or sex often fill. You and your child must be creative in finding those activities, events, or hobbies that are rewarding to *your* child. In Exercise 22, your child will list alternative ways of meeting his or her needs. Then you will brainstorm things to do to meet those needs instead of using drugs or engaging in sex.

The possibilities are endless, so let your imaginations wander. There may be some things you have never tried before that you think might be rewarding or fun. Be creative! At the end of the

---

Exercise 22   **PARENT and CHILD**

FINDING ALTERNATIVES

Note: This activity involves both parents and their children, but instructions are directed to the child.

The following list contains six major categories of needs that all people have in their lives. Circle one or two needs that are particularly important to you. If you think of another need that is important, write it in the list.

NEEDS: Social acceptance   Pleasure seeking
        Self-esteem enhancement   Escape
        Stress reduction   Risk taking
        Other _____

Write the need(s) in the spaces provided in the sentence below. Then make a list of ways to meet these needs.

These are things I could do to meet my needs for (1) _____
_____ and (2) _____

Need 1: _____   Need 2: _____

_____   _____
_____   _____
_____   _____
_____   _____
_____   _____
_____   _____

Now go back over the list and choose which things you would like to do most and which ones would be acceptable to both you and your parents. Think of ways you could actually make them happen. Then fill in the following sentence as though you were talking to your parents.

I would really like to _____, and
you could help me do this by _____
_____

Parents: Your child has listed several ways to meet important needs in his or her life. Can you or will you help make these happen? (Yes or No) If so, how are you willing to help? _____
_____

chapter there's a list of alternative activities generated by groups of teenagers. If you get stuck, you may want to refer to that list, but the best solutions are always the ones you and your child come up with. After all, you know best what meets your own needs. By fulfilling needs in acceptable ways, you may be helping to prevent the onset of unacceptable behaviors.

Get Involved in Alternatives

Some of the alternative activities your child has listed will require your time, permission, or financial resources. As a parent, you will need to make a commitment to help your child get involved in those activities that can help her stay away from drugs or sex. Make the alternatives you both discovered a priority for you. Be alert to other opportunities available in your community and encourage your child to get involved (i.e., Scouts, dance, sports, volunteer work, church groups, etc.).

Maybe an alternative of interest to your child is to "go hiking." If so, set a date and plan your hike. You may even want to go with your child and get to know him a little better. Don't just complete the exercises and not follow through with the alternatives. This will only prove disappointing to your child. Instead, *make them happen* by setting a time to do them.

Some of the alternatives your child has selected may not be feasible or possible, and it is important to acknowledge this to your child. Some may be undesirable to you, but be as flexible as you can. Your child may feel a need to do some things you don't want her to do; an undesirable alternative on the list may still be better than if she were to choose to take drugs or engage in inappropriate sexual behavior.

As a parent it is important that you let your child know that there are many alternatives in his life. Pursuing these alternatives gives children a sense of accomplishment and confidence in their abilities to try new things. The world knows you by what you do. Most teenagers want to be known for their accomplishments and their potentials, not for using drugs or being sexually active. Let your child know that these negative labels can stick with him (for example, "he's a druggie," "she's sleazy"), and that being known for other things is much more rewarding ("he's a good photographer," "she's quite an athlete"). As a parent, you may need to help your child pursue those goals that will meet her needs and give her the kind of recognition and acknowledgement you both can live with.

LIST OF ALTERNATIVES

Social Needs

Meet new people
Call a friend on the phone
Join a club
Go dancing
Go on a picnic
Have a party
Go to an amusement park
Share secrets with a friend
Go on a date
Introduce yourself to
   someone new
Invite someone to your
   house

Pleasure-Seeking Needs

Play any sport
Dance
Act silly
Fly a kite
Listen to music
Go sailing
Skateboard
Play arcade games
Eat sweets
Play with animals
Travel
Get a massage
Go to a restaurant
Help someone else
Sunbathe
Play ping-pong
Hug someone

(continued)

(*LIST OF ALTERNATIVES, continued*)

Self-Esteem Needs

Get in shape
Sing songs
Have your hair cut
Take up a new hobby
Get a facial or a manicure
Take care of a pet
Volunteer time at a hospital
Buy a special outfit
Do something you're good at
List things to do; get them
    done
Talk with a special friend
Tell yourself three things
    you like about yourself
Ask others what they like
    about you

Stress Reduction Needs

Go swimming
Meditate
Listen to music
Do aerobic exercises
Go sailing
Watch TV
Take a hot bath or jacuzzi
Go fishing
Lay on the grass and look
    at the sky
Daydream
Take a nap
Ride a bike
Get a massage
Sunbathe

Escape Needs

Go shopping
Watch a movie
Listen to music
Go hiking
Watch TV
Read a book
Take a nap
Go fishing
Take a day trip
Go to a museum
Take a long walk
Write a letter
Go camping

Risk-Taking Needs

Fly in a plane
Race bicycles
Ride a motorcycle
Go sailing
Climb mountains
Go canoeing
Camp out overnight in
the
    woods
Go skiing
Travel
Hold a séance
Skateboard or roller
skate
Dive off the high dive
Ride a roller coaster
Introduce yourself to
    someone new
Play football

10

DECISIONS, DECISIONS, DECISIONS

The decisions your child makes—whether or not to take drugs or have sex—could have a profound impact on his life, both now and in the future. Parents teach their children many skills to help them through life, but rarely do they teach their children how to go about making good decisions. How *do* you make decisions?

Decisions are part of everyone's life. We make hundreds of decisions each day, some with careful thought and some without a moment's hesitation. We must decide whether to get up when the alarm clock sounds or go back to sleep. We must decide which clothes to wear, whether to shower before or after breakfast, which route to take to work, and what to eat for lunch. We must decide how to approach an assignment, whether or not to remind our kid to clean his room, what to watch on TV, how much salt to add to the sauce. . . . the list goes on. Often these *daily decisions* seem to happen almost automatically.

By contrast, *future decisions* are the kinds of decisions that pave the way for the direction our lives may take or the outcomes we may face. They include such decisions as what courses to take in school, what career to pursue, what to do in case the house catches fire, how to react when a neighbor asks to borrow the lawn mower for the hundredth time, what to pack for a camping trip, who to marry, where to live, and so on. These decisions are attempts to anticipate, and prepare for, the future.

Deciding not to Decide

Future decisions often seem more difficult to make than daily decisions because the need to make them is usually not so immediate and because the outcome of the decision is usually more important. These decisions often require a commitment to a particular course in life, and, for this reason, we put them off until the right solution comes along or until we can wait no longer. This is known as the "Scarlett O'Hara" method of decision making, or the "I'll think about it tomorrow" approach. The important thing to acknowledge is that putting off a decision is, in itself, a decision. It is deciding not to decide.

Active Decision Making

A person who takes an active role in making future decisions has more control over the future because he is prepared for the possibilities that may arise. For this reason, it is important that children begin to make decisions *now* about drug use and sex. Leaving these decisions until the "situation arises" may mean that your child has to make a hasty choice amidst great peer pressure about a very important aspect of his life.

There are several myths about decision making that should be clarified.

Myth: Children are born with the innate "common sense" to make decisions rationally.

Fact: The ability to make decisions is a skill that is learned, and one which can be greatly improved with education, modeling, and practice.

Myth: There is always one, and only one, right decision.

Fact: There are always many choices with many possible outcomes; more than one choice (or maybe no choices) will work out well.

Myth: Once a decision has been made it shouldn't be changed, so you should take lots of time making that decision.

Fact: Many decisions can be changed. Sometimes just making a decision and acting on it gives you more information about the problem, which may help you make a better decision.

It is important that your child make an *active* decision about drugs and sex and that she has the *decision-making skills* to do so.

Decision-Making Skills

There are five steps involved in good decision making. Each step is critical.

1. Identify the problem
2. List all options
3. Specify the possible outcomes of each option
4. Review the outcomes and select the best option
5. Act on that decision

Identify the Problem

Before you can start to make a decision, you must clarify what the problem really is, or what question you are asking yourself. Vague problems often defeat the decision-making process because they make your choices hazy. For example, the problem of "I'm not happy these days" is much too nebulous. It must be further refined by asking questions of yourself to pinpoint the main problem to be solved or decision to be made.

You might start by asking "What parts of my life make me unhappy" and learn that it is your job. Then you could further refine the problem by exploring just exactly what it is about your job that you don't like, and you may, as an example, realize that you can't seem to get along with your boss. Now you're getting somewhere. You have narrowed the problem to something you can put your finger on, and you can begin to think of ways of dealing with that problem.

List All Options

When faced with a problem, people often make decisions based on the first option that comes to them or the option that they have

129

used most often in the past. This limits the options available to you and may lead you to overlook perfectly good options that might solve the problem. This method of decision making is not only unsophisticated, it also increases the chances of making the same mistakes over and over because you have not spent time thinking of other alternatives.

In this stage of decision making, it is important to "brainstorm" all possible options. Let your mind be as open as possible and do not censor any options just yet. That comes later. Write down all the options you think of on a piece of paper, one option on each line, to form a column. Since this stage is the one that defines the range of possible decisions you might' make, it is important to spend lots of time on it. Do not dismiss anything as "silly" just yet and try to be as creative as possible in coming up with options.

For example, if the problem is that you don't get along with your boss, your options might be: quit the job, kill the boss, do nice things for your boss so he'll like you, find out what your boss expects of your work and do it, talk to the boss and try to settle your differences, transfer to another department, fake an illness and try to get disability, or conspire with your colleagues and try to get your boss fired by his boss. A few of these options might be ludicrous and may even cause you to laugh out loud, but don't stop the thinking process by taking time to censor those options.

Specify the Outcomes

Now it's time to look at the positive and negative outcomes that are likely to accompany each of the options. To simplify this process, you might want to eliminate any options that are impossible, impractical, or unethical. In the example above, you might want to eliminate "kill the boss," "fake an illness," and "conspire with colleagues." Do not eliminate options just yet unless you are *really* sure they are not options. With some exploration, some seemingly lousy options can look better and better.

Next to your list of options make two columns, one for "positive outcomes" and one for "negative outcomes" (see sample). Consider each option separately and devote enough time to

Sample

DECISION-MAKING WORKSHEET

Step 1—*Identify the Problem*

Problem: I am unhappy with my job because I can't get along with my boss.

Steps 2 and 3—*List All Options and Specify the Outcomes*

	Outcomes	
Options	**Positive**	**Negative**
transfer to another department	—more supportive boss —new tasks —better office —new colleagues	—not enough training —lose seniority —new colleagues —can't leave at 4:00 —miss friends —"quitter"
find out what boss expects and do it	—keep job —know what's expected —better relationship with boss	—get more work —can't do what's expected
quit job	etc.	etc.
kill boss		
try to settle diff's		
fake an illness and get disability		
get boss fired		

Step 4—*Circle the Important Outcomes and Make a Decision*

Important Outcomes: keeping job and seniority; good relationships with boss and co-workers

Decision: Find out what the boss expects and do it.

Step 5—*Act on the Decision*

Plan of Action: Make an appointment with the boss this week to discuss the problem and find out what he expects of me.

thoroughly assess the positive and negative outcomes that are likely to happen if you decided on that option. Be realistic in your assessments—a test of your assessments might be "would most people agree that this outcome would happen?"

In the columns next to each option, write down the positive and negative outcomes you have identified. Only when you have exhausted your outcomes should you move on to the next option. When you have finished writing the outcomes for each option, go back and see if there are any important ones you might have overlooked or forgotten.

In the example of the disagreeable boss, the positive outcomes of the option to transfer to another department might include: a more supportive boss, exciting new tasks, a better office, meeting new people. The negative outcomes might include: not having the training to do the job well, losing seniority, having to learn how to work with new colleagues, a boss who won't let you leave at 4:00 on Friday, not seeing your friends in the present office very often, being labeled by the company as "uncooperative" or as a "quitter."

Review the Outcomes and Select the Best Option

Now that all the positive and negative outcomes have been noted, it is time to make use of them. As you will notice, some outcomes seem more important to you than others. Review the outcomes in each column and circle those that are the most important to you. In the example above, if a challenging job is important, the outcome of "exciting new tasks" might be circled. Or if it is crucial that you leave by 4:00 on Fridays to make your long-standing racquetball match, then that option should be circled.

The importance of each outcome depends on what *you* value, and the most important outcomes should weigh more heavily in your decision. Try not to circle so many outcomes that you become overwhelmed by the importance of them all, nor too few that you lose sight of the true benefits and risks of choosing a given option.

Now step back from your worksheet. You may even want to take a break to gain a different perspective. Review the outcomes of each option and make a decision based on those outcomes. The best option is usually the one with the most positive outcomes, particularly if many of the positive outcomes but few of the negative outcomes are circled.

If two options seem equally attractive, select one with the understanding that you may resort to the other later if circumstances permit. If no options seem attractive, select the least objectional option and make a commitment to reevaluate your situation later.

Before making a final decision about an option, look at the most negative outcome of that option and ask yourself, "Could I live with this?" If you cannot truly live with that outcome, you should not make that decision. For example, if "go to jail" were an outcome of the option to "kill the boss," and you could not live with that outcome, then "kill the boss" ceases to be an option.

Act on the Decision

By this stage, you have used your decision-making skills to determine the best option, and it is now time to act on that decision. Don't "second guess" yourself by ruminating about whether or not your decision is the best one, or whether or not it will work. The only way to really find out is to enact that decision. Taking action is important because it circumvents the natural tendencies to procrastinate when faced with tough decisions.

Taking action on your decision also gives you a chance to test out your hypotheses about the outcomes of that decision. In the preceding example of the disagreeable boss, the decision might have been to "find out what the boss expects of your work and do it." Maybe one of your anticipated negative outcomes of that option was "the boss will give me too much work." When you act on your decision and approach the boss, he says to you, "I always thought you were goofing off, but now that I have reviewed your work I see that you have many more responsibilities than I realized." Instead of giving you more work, your workload stays the same and the boss has increased admiration for your performance.

In this case, the anticipated negative outcome did not happen, and the decision turned out to be a good one. Sometimes the outcomes might be different, and might even be *more* negative than you anticipated. The point is, you will never know the true outcomes until you *act on your decision.*

Don't be fooled by the myth that "once you make a decision it can't be changed." Indeed, acting on a decision usually gives you more information to use if you need to change your decision. If your decision still doesn't solve the problem, start again with the decision-making steps. This time you'll have more information to add to your lists of outcomes, and you'll be able to omit some of the options you have already tried. Whenever you begin the process of making a decision, do so with a commitment to act on that decision. Otherwise, the process becomes merely an exercise in futility.

Making Decisions About Drugs and Sex

It is important for youngsters to make decisions now about drugs and sex so that they will have time to consider all possible options and outcomes and be prepared with a decision when faced with the actual problem. As parents, you can be particularly helpful in this decision-making process if you follow a few guidelines.

1. Be a resource for your child. Point out *realistic* outcomes of using drugs or engaging in sex. Be sure to include outcomes that can occur at the time of the behavior (such as getting sick while drinking) as well as those that can happen in the future (becoming an alcoholic). Be informed.
2. Encourage your *child* to give examples of outcomes. This will have a much greater impact on her behavior than if you simply tell her about the outcomes.
3. Be believable. Do not exaggerate negative outcomes or minimize positive ones. Propaganda on the evils of sex or drugs, like the film *Reefer Madness,* tends to backfire and may actually encourage kids to try the behaviors. Similarly, discounting the positive effects of drugs or sex will limit your credibility.
4. Do not force your decision on your child. Chances are good that it will not be acted upon and it may be reacted against. Help your child come to his own decision and support his ability to use the decision-making skills.

PRACTICE MAKING DECISIONS

Using the steps listed in this chapter, practice decision-making skills with your child. The Decision-Making Worksheet at the back of this chapter (page 143) will give you the format for recording each step. Make a copy of the worksheet and use it to help you complete the following exercise.

Choose a problem that is interesting to you and your child, preferably one that is not too emotion-laden for the two of you. Solicit your child's input in selecting a topic.

Some suggestions:

- Where should the family go on vacation?
- How should we cope with a family illness?
- How could we plan our routines so that we can spend some time together as a family?
- When should we buy a new car and what kind should we buy?
- Select any current problem or question facing your family.

Follow the steps outlined in this chapter when filling out the worksheet. The example on page 136 shows how one family made a decision about "Where to go on vacation" by using the worksheet. You may want to review this with your child before starting on your own worksheet so that you can familiarize your child with the decision-making process.

When you have finished, evaluate your decision-making skills by answering the following questions:

1. Did you spend enough time listing the options or are there more you didn't consider?

2. Did you list realistic positive and negative outcomes for each option?

3. Were you able to avoid making up your mind too quickly? (For example, did you weigh each option separately and fairly without favoring one from the start?)

4. Did you circle your most important outcomes and weigh them more heavily when deciding?

5. How good do you think your decision was?

DECISION-MAKING EXAMPLE

Problem: Where should the family go for a two-week vacation this summer?

Options	Outcomes	
	Positive	**Negative**
1) Go to grandparents' house	relaxing inexpensive	boring—no friends nothing new to see just saw them two months ago
2) Go to Disneyland	exciting trip something new fun for everyone in family nice weather beaches nearby	have to fly there stay in hotel have to rent car
3) Go camping in Yellowstone National Park	could drive there exciting trip something new hiking camping could bring a friend along moderate expense	it might rain around each other the whole time get pretty dirty long drive
4) Rent a cabin at the lake	relaxing short drive swimming, boating, fishing moderate expense could bring a friend along	nothing new to see it might rain could get boring

Important Outcomes: Have to watch the budget and want to go someplace exciting that we have never seen before.

Decision: Family will go to Yellowstone.

Plan of Action: We will go for two weeks in May, and Jennie can bring a friend with her. Dad will make reservations and organize camping gear. Mom will organize food stuffs. Jennie will look up information in the library about Yellowstone.

5. Do not omit options simply because they are repellent to you. In every case, there is always the option to use drugs or engage in sex; it is crucial that your child consider the positive and negative outcomes of these options. Ignoring these options does not make them go away . . . it just makes them mysterious.

6. As part of specifying the outcomes, *occasionally* point out what your reaction would be if your child were to choose a particular option. Try not to be overly punitive as this might squelch open communication. Do not, for example, threaten to disinherit your child if he uses marijuana, or the exercise will most likely come to a halt. On the other hand, if you would be disappointed in your child for using marijuana, or if you would seek professional help, let him know this when the option of using marijuana is entertained. Keep your messages as matter-of-fact as possible and don't give too many of them. Your child will get the message that there are outcomes that will come from you and that these too should be considered as *part* of the decision-making process.

The next exercise presents problems related to drugs or sex that most teenagers face at some point in their lives. You and your child will be asked to complete a Decision-Making Worksheet on each of the problems presented. The following example may help show you how to complete the exercise.

Example

Margie and her mother worked together, using the Decision-Making Worksheet, to deal with the following problem:

Your friend invited you over on your birthday and when you arrived, you found out it was a surprise party for you! Your friend had also invited a cute guy that you secretly liked and wanted to get to know better. Several people brought presents for you and when you opened one, you found a joint of marijuana. The person who gave it to you said, jokingly, "Happy birthday. I guess you're old enough to smoke this now."

They discussed the situation and Margie was able to define the problem more specifically.

Problem: What should I do with the joint?

Then Margie and her mother listed several possible options and came up with positive and negative outcomes of each. (Three options are shown below as examples.) Margie's Mom let her think of most of the outcomes and she added some suggestions when Margie got stuck. This is what they came up with:

Options	Outcomes	
	Positive	**Negative**
1) Accept it and share it with others	Get high Others might enjoy Feel older Relax more	Bad reputation with guy Friends think I use Get caught and punished Bad effect on lungs Get in accident Act stupid and silly
2) Give it back to the person	Feel confident Impress guy Be myself Not endanger health	Look like a nerd Friends who smoke might avoid me Seem ungrateful
3) Say "thanks" and secretly flush it down the toilet	More discrete Seem cool	Friends think I'm stingy Guy thinks I use pot Will be faced with this decision again Didn't stand up for myself

After reviewing the options and outcomes, Margie circled several that were important to her and wrote them down.

Important Outcomes: Impress the guy I like, respect for myself, keep my friends' respect

She saw that most of the important positive outcomes went with Option 2. The important negative outcomes seemed to go with

138

Options 1 and 3. Margie made a decision and wrote down a plan of action.

Decision: Option 2—Give the joint back to the person.

Plan of Action: In the event that something like this should happen to me, I will give the joint back to the person. I wouldn't want that guy or my friends to think of me as a pot smoker, and I would want to stand up for myself.

Now it's your turn. Using the Decision-Making Worksheet on page 143 (make four copies), you and your child must decide how to handle the four problems listed in Exercise 24. The exercise will help your child develop his decision-making skills and will insure that he has considered many of the outcomes that might occur if he were to choose to use drugs or engage in sex. Be sure to look at the Appendix if you need more information. Also, refer to your child's list of reasons for not using drugs or having sex from Exercise 21 in the previous chapter.

This exercise need not be completed in a single session. It may help to spread it out over several discussions so your child will not be inundated with too much decision making. When you begin your decision-making worksheets, be sure to describe the problem as you see it. Then list *all* the options you can think of, even if you know you wouldn't choose some of them. Youngsters should be encouraged to list the outcomes first with little input from parents. Then parents can comment on the outcomes, clarifying and/or enhancing the list. Be sure the outcomes include things that might happen *right away* as well as *in the future.* (For example, with cigarette smoking, your breath and clothes would smell right away and you might get lung cancer in the future.)

By helping your child deal with the hypothetical problem situations, you force him to put himself in that situation and think about the consequences of his actions and the numerous options that are available to him. Let your child know that he can direct his own future in many ways by considering lots of options and making active decisions.

Recent reports indicate that girls who are most likely to become pregnant are those who see little opportunity in their future.

Exercise 24	PARENT and CHILD

DECISION-MAKING PROBLEMS

Using four copies of the Decision-Making Worksheet, you and your child will work together to make decisions about what to do in the following problem situations.

Problem 1—Your boyfriend/girlfriend has asked you to come over while his/her parents are out of town. He/she would like your relationship to become more intimate and sexual, and feels that it is time that the two of you either had sex or started to cool off the relationship and date other people. You really like this person a lot and don't want to end the relationship.

Problem 2—Your friend smokes cigarettes and suggests that you should at least practice smoking so that you don't look like a nerd when the rest of the group is smoking.

Problem 3—You have just been invited to a party this weekend and all your friends will be going. You know there's going to be a lot of drinking, because you heard one guy say he was getting a keg of beer.

Problem 4—You and some friends are listening to music and one friend suggests that marijuana makes music sound better. Someone lights up a joint and it is passed around the circle to you.

Children who feel that the future looks bleak and who believe that their options are limited are much more likely to turn to drugs and sex to provide pleasure in the present. As the previous chapter on "Finding Alternatives" suggests, there are many options and alternatives in life and it is important that you help your child discover them.

Just as you need to help your child explore new options and alternatives to drugs and sex, it is important to point out the negative outcomes of engaging in those behaviors. Find out what your child's future goals and dreams are and help her to see how drug use and inappropriate sexual behavior can interfere with those goals.

The young woman with dreams of going to college may be forced to reconsider her dreams if her sexual activities result in pregnancy. The young man who loses his driver's license for driving under the influence of alcohol won't be able to return to his summer job driving a delivery truck. Know your child's goals and emphasize the importance of considering the future when making decisions about drugs and sex.

Keeping Your Skills Tuned

The ability to make good decisions and analyze options well depends on practicing these skills often. Parents should encourage their children to participate actively in everyday decisions. Parents should also use the skills themselves and provide good role models for how to make decisions.

Use daily problems as your practice field. With something as simple as deciding which fast food place to visit, enumerate the options out loud and discuss the positive and negative outcomes of each. Is one closer? Is one less expensive? Does one have the best french fries while another has the best burgers? Which gives faster service? Then think about which outcomes or factors are the most important to you right now (maybe you're really in the mood for some good french fries), weigh the outcomes, and decide where to go. This need only take a few minutes, but it reinforces your child's decision-making skills.

As another example, if you are planning on buying a major item such as a car, let your child in on the decision-making process. List the cars that are options and the positive and negative outcomes associated with each. These might include price, appearance, maintenance record, size, mileage, and other factors. Ask your child to give input throughout the decision-making process and encourage sensible suggestions and comments. This will increase your child's confidence in making decisions.

It is important to practice decision-making skills, but it is also important to do so in moderation. Do not make every problem a "major decision" or you may spoil the spontaneity and fun of making some spur-of-the-moment choices. Just be sure that important decisions are made with adequate deliberation and not left to chance.

Not every decision needs to be bogged down with lists. At first, the worksheets help to refine the skills, but with time and practice the skills become automatic. Thinking of a variety of options will become second nature; considering the positive and negative outcomes will become standard procedure. Give your child a little room to make his own decisions so that through trial and error he will learn how to perfect this skill. You have had many years of practice, and it is crucial that your child practice too . . . particularly while he can still rely on you for guidance.

DECISION-MAKING WORKSHEET

Problem:

Options	Outcomes	
	Positive	**Negative**

(Continue on a separate sheet of paper if necessary)

Importance Outcomes: (List and circle above)

Decision:

Plan of Action:

11

IT'S IN YOUR HANDS

As a parent, you can wield a great deal of power in getting others to do something about kids, drugs, and sex. Other parents will listen to you. The schools will listen to you. Your community will listen to you. And when parents, schools, and the community at large are all saying the same thing, you can bet that young people will listen to you too.

It is time to stop investing your energies exclusively in your own nuclear family. Work with others. The effort that it takes to build a coalition of concerned members can pay off in a healthier environment for your family and neighbors.

Wringing Hands (recognizing the problem)

What prompts parents and school systems to set up programs to reduce drug use and teen pregnancy? It may be a reaction to an existing problem, such as a high rate of pregnancy among high school girls or a high rate of drug abuse among high school boys. On the other hand, it may be a reaction to a headline about a drug bust or a serious car accident involving drunken adolescent party-goers.

Holding Hands (finding others to join in)

Facing problems or potential problems alone can sometimes be a formidable task. There is strength in numbers—support, ideas, resources, a united message to young people.

Start with other parents you know, with your child's teacher, with the school principal, with the Parent-Teacher Association.

Do not forget the churches, civic groups, health services, and others. You will find that you are not alone in feeling concerned. Your feelings will also be shared by many young people, so do not leave them out of your network. *Start your own group* by setting a time to meet with others to discuss the problems.

Let Your Fingers Do the Walking (find out more about the problem)

Learn more about drug use and teen sexuality—not only about the extent of the problem, but also about the success of different approaches to the problems. Contact local and national resources. Read the literature. Talk to local experts who have been involved in prevention programs or who can refer you to someone who has. Other parent groups and school systems are more than willing to share their experiences. You can begin your research by checking with some of the resources listed in Appendix D.

Show of Hands (decide what to do)

Doing something about the problem begins with the question of what to do and where to start. Prioritize your goals as a group and start to work on one or two at a time. In any collaborative effort, there will be different opinions; it is important to respect others' opinions even though they differ from your own. When individuals fight over personal agendas, the program will either stall or never even get going. Use your collective energies to act, not to debate HOW to act.

Helping Hands (becoming an active program)

Put your plans into action. Be flexible, yet try to maintain a clear sense of where you are going. It helps to divide a goal into a series of steps and then delegate responsibilities for accomplishing these steps to several group members. Active involvement keeps people interested and committed. Try to delegate responsibilities that will lead to success by focusing on your easier goals; leave the tougher challenges for later. For example, your group's goal may be to close down the liquor store near the school. A first step may be to increase parent awareness that the liquor store presents a problem. A second step may be to find out the mechanism

145

for changing zoning ordinances. A third step could involve starting a petition. Once these steps are sure of success, then the more challenging steps of persuading the store owner to move or preparing for a hearing by the zoning board could begin.

Basic Approaches to School-Based Curricula

Many schools already have drug prevention programs; some have sex education courses. These range from one or two lectures in class to a complete course or semester on drug prevention or sex education. The expertise of the teachers likewise ranges widely, from teachers with little formal training who may use no materials or materials from community agencies, to teachers who have been specially trained in drug prevention or sex education techniques.

Any program you may wish to have your school undertake should take more than one of the following approaches:

Factual Information

Too many young people base their decisions on myths and misinformation. For example, many girls have become pregnant because they thought they couldn't get pregnant if they had sex standing up, if it was their first time, if they douched afterward, and so on. Other youngsters may try marijuana thinking it is harmless or not realizing that the drug may be laced with a more potent and hazardous drug, such as PCP. Straight facts about drugs and sex can better lead a young person to making good lifestyle decisions.

Instilling Self-Esteem

If we value who we are, we are less likely to jeopardize ourselves. For those youngsters who may use drugs or engage in sex (or get pregnant) in order to feel important, a program that instills self-esteem can minimize the need for escape. Feeling good about ourselves means we don't need a crutch, we can dare to hold fast to what we believe, and we can have faith in the values we are developing for ourselves.

146

Decision Making

As children reach their teen years, they begin to understand the concept of consequences. Being young, they have not developed their decision-making skills enough to consider those consequences beyond the immediate intent to feel good or try an adult behavior. By learning decision-making skills, children can look at the larger picture and evaluate the future consequences of their behaviors before acting.

Role Modeling

Many programs train peer leaders to serve as role models for refusing drugs or sexual advances. Some also use peers as counselors for teens who have problems or questions. Adolescents are more likely to trust and open up to someone who is like them.

Peer Pressure Resistance

How does a young person say NO to peers without losing face, being pressured against his or her decision, or fearing negative consequences? Holding realistic discussions and practicing how to say NO have shown to be successful techniques for drug prevention. These same skills can help the young person who does not want to have sex.

A Well-Rounded Support System is Crucial

Providing teens with a good classroom program is not enough to solve the problem. A strong school program must be supported by administrators, school policies, and parents.

School administrators not only have to support the concept that drug or pregnancy prevention is critical, they must also be supportive of the time it takes for teacher preparation and in the allocation of class time and expenses for needed materials.They must further welcome the active participation of parents.

School drug policies must create a school climate prohibiting use, possession, and sale of drugs. Rules regarding social conduct should encourage respect toward others and insist upon chaperoned school events. The policies must be clear, visibly communicated, and consistently enforced. Read that last sentence again; it is the key to a strong and successful school policy and is too often overlooked.

Parental support comes in the form of good role modeling, vocal support of school programs and policies, and active participation. At home, you should let your child know that you agree with the school's efforts; supplement the school program with your own family discussions or with exercises such as those found in this book.

It is important for all involved to understand that issues such as drug use and sexuality must be shaped within a child's family, where she will learn morals and values, and echoed in her primary social setting, the school, where she obtains most of her away-from-home influences. Consider the magnitude of what you want to achieve. Is it realistic to expect one course about drugs or sex to change a student's behavior? Other school subjects are geared toward the goals of increasing knowledge or possibly influencing attitudes. It is much easier to reach these goals than to actually influence a behavior.

Behavior change has been achieved in a number of drug education programs studied throughout the nation. Research has shown that a carefully planned program of skill practice, information exchange, and discussion, along with techniques such as writing out contracts for avoiding drugs and listing a personal set of reasons for not using drugs, can prevent the grade-school student from trying or abusing substances.

Sex education has not been researched to the same degree. One reason is that only a small percentage of schools have actually offered model programs to students. Those studies that have been conducted show that sex education can have a positive effect and can postpone the age at which a young person engages in intercourse.

Most students are ignorant of reproduction and contraception. Many become pregnant because of misinformation leading them to believe that they cannot or will not become pregnant. Sex education has clearly shown that it can increase knowledge. Moreover, young people who have participated in a sex education program that discusses contraception are more apt to use protection when they do become sexually active.

A school program or any formal program that includes parent and child interaction at home can be quite successful. Both parents and children report side benefits, such as increased communication. Parents can activate school programs by vocalizing their interest. Schools respond to the demands of parents, so use your clout.

Schools Take Action!

So you are ready to launch a school program, either a new one or a more effective modification of an existing one. Here are some basic steps to follow:

1. Help to establish school policies on acceptable social behavior. Teachers, students, school administrators, and parents should establish and implement the policies as a team.

2. Provide training to teachers who are truly interested in teaching students about drugs and teen sexuality.

3. Promote the importance of having a healthy lifestyle at school and at home. Use posters, distribute interesting literature, include the message in discussions and conversations, invite speakers, and so on.

4. Chaperone social functions, both on and off school grounds.

5. Make available current resource materials: library books, magazines, pamphlets, audiovisual materials.

6. Support parent networks and become actively involved.

7. Support student groups that engage in activities that provide alternatives to drug use and sex.

8. Invite outside speakers such as parents, experts, and others to talk to students; this helps make your messages relevant outside the classroom.

9. Evaluate your program to see if it works. Don't just assume that it is effective. Always be on the lookout for new information on effective school programs and techniques.

Basic Approaches of Parent Groups

Parent groups across the country have been started by people just like you. Perhaps the most basic principle underlying the parent groups is one of caring. All you need is to care that your child will grow up healthy and strong. You do not need to know all about drugs or teenage sexuality—that knowledge can be learned along the way. You do not need to feel completely comfortable talking about these subjects with your child—that comfortableness will come as you open the lines of communications.

Parents will choose for themselves what they want their groups to accomplish. Some of the more basic approaches include the following:

Communication

As a first step, remove the heavy burden of expecting your child to read your mind. A clear message from you that is echoed by other parents in your group helps set norms for acceptable behavior. The mere fact that you are part of a concerned parents' group is a strong message in itself.

Enforcement

As a parent, you cannot be everywhere at all times. What a comfort it is to know that other parents agree to chaperone their own children's parties, set appropriate curfews, refuse to permit their children to use drugs or alcohol, expect an appropriate level of sexual behavior and respect for the opposite sex, and will expect from your child when he is visiting the same standard of conduct that you would expect.

Role Modeling

Your actions and the actions of other adults can speak louder than words. Although adults hesitate to comment upon how others

150

should behave, it is reasonable to request that parents within the group try hard to provide an example of responsible adult behavior. It is not necessary to develop a standard of conduct; most parents respond positively when they realize how strong an influence their own behaviors can have on youngsters.

Skill Building

Every parent has a great deal they can teach their children: decision making, holding fast to one's values, learning to resist temptations and pressures, and so on. Your parent group may wish to ask for guidance in imparting these skills or hold group sessions on each of these areas that include children as well as parents.

Community Action

Get involved in your community. Work to build a community climate that encourages the young to make healthy choices. Ask the police to enforce laws and regulations more strictly. Ask them to notify parents of a young person who has committed an offense. Encourage the judicial system to prosecute offenders appropriately and to send out the message that irresponsibility can have legal consequences. Approach merchants about making drugs, alcohol, and cigarettes less available. Ask them to make contraceptives more available. Devise education and counseling services for the young through mental health centers, hospitals, schools, youth organizations, and so on.

Parents Take Action!

Parent groups are for parents, therefore few rules exist outside of knowing how to work together. There are, however, some basic tips that can help you conduct a successful group:

1. Simply get started. How or why doesn't matter nearly so much as merely taking that first step.

2. Set some objectives for the group. Nothing fails so quickly as a group without direction or activity. Objectives can

range from just listening to one another's concerns about setting uniform standards of conduct, such as curfews, to receiving and providing training for parents interested in knowing more about drugs and teen sexuality.

3. Meet regularly and keep a commitment to do so.

4. Maintain a comfortable and friendly atmosphere.

5. Select leaders who can be responsible for administrative and management needs. It is important to have at least one committed parent who will keep the ball rolling even if others drop out.

6. Invite experts to come speak with you. Share your own expertise, knowledge acquired from reading, and personal family experiences.

7. Take it home. Don't spend your assertiveness, concern, good ideas, and communication skills just in the parent group—it belongs at home with your children.

8. Be creative. Use common sense. These are the two most critical dynamics for a successful parent group.

9. Join in with other efforts in schools, churches, civic organizations, youth groups, and elsewhere.

12

BEYOND PREVENTION

How can you tell if your son is using drugs? How can you tell if your daughter is sexually active? There are many signs that can give you a clue about your child's behavior. The key to understanding what is going on with your child is to look for *changes* in behavior and *patterns* of signs that point to a problem.

Ignoring the warning signs until the evidence is overwhelming can allow a problem to get out of hand. Parents often have a need to believe that "my child would never do that," and they may choose to overlook facts that suggest otherwise. On the other hand, reading too much into any one sign may give parents a distorted picture. When looked at individually, many of the signs of drug use or sexual activity are also signs of natural adolescent development. For example, it is natural for an adolescent to want to spend more time alone, maybe sitting in his room listening to music. A pattern of repeated avoidance of family members, a decline in school performance, frequent curfew violations, and an increased use of eyedrops may, however, indicate a more serious problem. *Look for patterns.*

What are the signs? The lists below present some behavioral and physical signs that might indicate drug use or sexual activity. Bear in mind that the use of alcohol and nicotine (cigarettes) is considered drug use, and that the use of these substances can set the stage for using "hard drugs" later.

Signs of Drug Use

Behavioral Signs

School performance declines: lower grades, decreased attendance or unexcused absences, homework not completed, concerns expressed by teachers

Behavior around friends changes: more secretive, chooses friends who have reputations for using drugs, talks or jokes about drugs around friends

Commitments are not kept: comes home late, lies about where he is going, doesn't complete responsibilities at home

Increased use of eyedrops, nasal spray, breath spray or mints

Avoids parents/family: withdraws into bedroom, won't make eye contact, spends less and less time with family

Alcohol, cigarettes, prescription drugs, or money are missing from home

Possesses drug paraphernalia: cigarette papers, "roach clips," tiny spoons, tiny vials, cigarettes, lighter, pipes or other smoking apparatus, small straws or rolled up bills, bottle opener or corkscrew, etc.

Changes in thought processes: decreased attention span, easily distracted, forgetful, lack of motivation, slow to understand what is said

Trouble with authorities: legal violations, breaking school rules, lying to parents or other adults

Increased irritability or argumentativeness

Physical Signs

Bloodshot or watery eyes, pupils unusually dilated or constricted, vacant stare

Persistent flulike or coldlike symptoms: runny nose, cough

Odors present on breath or clothes: tobacco, alcohol, marijuana

Nervousness or jitteriness

Sensitivity to strong light or noise (hangover)

Marked change in activity, either overly active or lethargic

Changes in sleep patterns, either increased or decreased sleep

Changes in appetite: increased eating (especially junk food) or binge eating, decreased appetite, rapid weight loss or gain

Decreased concern for physical appearance or hygiene

Needle marks, often found on inside of elbow

Signs of drug use differ for the different drugs. Become familiar with drug effects so that you can understand what you're dealing with. These same symptoms may also be present when there are other physical or emotional illnesses. In either case, the cause of the symptoms needs to be investigated.

Signs of Sexual Activity

Behavioral Signs

Exclusive, long-term relationship
Many one-time-only dates, often made at the last minute
Secretiveness about dates
Lying about where s/he has been
Secretly arranging to be alone for extended period of time
Rumors about his/her sexual activity
Any indications of fears of pregnancy: unusual secretiveness or
  unwillingness to discuss menstrual periods, extreme nervous-
  ness around time of expected period
Staying out later than allowed, or out at odd hours
Skipping out of school with someone of opposite sex
Spending less time with same-sex friends; with opposite-sex
  friends almost all the time
Strong dependency on a relationship; sense of desperation and
  willingness to do anything to preserve that relationship
Sexist comments that suggest a lack of respect for the opposite
  sex

Physical Signs

Possession of birth control devices (pills, prophylactics, foam)
"Hickies" or bruise marks on the neck
Disheveled clothing after a date
Lost or found clothing, particularly intimate apparel
Any indications of pregnancy: morning sickness, missed periods,
  weight gain
Any indications of sexually transmitted disease: reports of painful
  urination, vaginal/penile itching or sores or unusual dis-
  charge

155

The signs noted above provide *possible* indicators of sexual activity. The determination of whether or not your child is sexually active, or, more importantly, whether he or she is *inappropriate* in his or her sexual behavior, must be determined by a closer examination of what is going on. Overlooking these signs because of embarrassment or unwillingness to see your child as a sexual being may lead to problems, such as teenage pregnancy or a sexually transmitted disease. On the other hand, being overly suspicious or using one sign as proof of promiscuity may serve to alienate you from your child by destroying trust.

Confronting Your Child

What do you do when you notice several signs of drug use or sexual behavior? You go right to the source and check it out—ask your child about it. The way you approach the situation will have a big effect on how it turns out, so a few words of caution are in order. Here are two styles used by many parents that often meet with failure:

1. The *heavy-handed* approach: This approach is characterized by anger and hostility on the part of the parent, which is soon mirrored in the child. It often begins with the parent "ambushing" the child unexpectedly, loudly accusing the child of being a "druggie" (or other term), throwing the evidence in the child's face, and demanding "What do you have to say for yourself?"

Parents may use this approach because their parents used it, or because they feel it will allow them to "catch my kid off guard so he'll be more likely to confess." In actuality, this approach promotes extreme defensiveness. If the child didn't do it, she will certainly lose trust in the parent. If she did do it, she may be so outraged or scared that she would not admit it. The parent and child become so polarized that neither can work toward resolving the problem and both feel a lot of resentment.

2. The *pussy-foot* approach: This approach is often used by a parent who suspects that his child is doing something wrong but (a) doesn't really want to know about it because then he would have to do something, (b) doesn't want to destroy the child's ten-

der ego, or (c) is too embarrassed to even talk about such topics as drugs or sex. Typically the approach is a vague and somewhat passive, "Is there something you want to tell me?" or "Is there something I should know?"

The subtle message this gives to a child is "I want to believe you are perfect so don't spoil it for me." The child who is in trouble and looking for help may be reluctant to disappoint his parents by telling the truth. Or he may be too embarrassed by the subject; his parent's own avoidance supports the belief that "you just don't talk about those kinds of things with your parents." The child who is in trouble and wants to hide it at all costs can get off easily with the simple answer, "Nothing's wrong." He knows his parents want to avoid the problem as much as he does.

Effective Confrontations

There are few things more frightening or disheartening as a parent than to suspect your child of drug abuse or inappropriate sexual behavior. The desire to know what is going on is equalled only by the fear of finding out the worst. It is not easy to confront your child, but it *is* necessary. It will undoubtedly feel uncomfortable both for you and your child, but do not let that stop you. Try to remain calm, open-minded, and empathic so that it will be easier for your child to tell the truth.

When confronting your child about possible drug abuse or sexual activity, it is important to . . .

- Convey an attitude of caring
- Present the evidence
- Seek outside information when necessary

The best approach is the direct, assertive approach with a genuine *attitude of caring*. Approach your child in a calm way. Let her know that you care about her and that you are concerned about her behavior. Acknowledge that you both may feel uncomfortable discussing the issue, but that it is important for you to understand what is happening.

Next, *present the evidence* that has come to your attention. If you

157

have found an empty beer bottle or a package of contraceptives, tell your child directly what you know. Do not withhold evidence in the hopes of gaining more information. You will lose trust. Tell your child what your fears are and ask him to explain the evidence. Ask questions if you need clarification.

If you are not satisfied that you have "the whole truth" despite your questioning, tell your child that you need to *seek outside information*. Let him help you determine who to ask to corroborate his story. If he is not cooperative, tell him how you plan to get the information you need and why it is important that you do so. Try to get the information in such a way that you can understand the extent of the problem (if any), yet avoid presenting your child as guilty or embarrassing him.

In the process of understanding your child's behavior, you may discover that the incident is a first-time offense or a relatively rare incident of experimentation. On the other hand, you may find out that it is a long-standing habit or problem that is more serious than you had imagined. The two situations call for different strategies.

Handling the First-Time Offender

If you are truly convinced that the "offense" does not represent a persistent behavior, you and your child can use this as a learning situation. It is important to understand why your child did what she did. It is also important to clarify exactly what you expect from her and which behaviors you will not tolerate.

There are four stages in confronting the first time offender:

1. *Understand why.* Try to get a clear understanding of what motivated your child to act in a certain way. Did she feel pressured to drink because everyone else was doing it? Did he seek sex in order to feel loved? Did she smoke pot out of curiosity? More importantly, get your child to look at why she did what she did. This may take some time and self-exploration to figure it out. There are always reasons behind actions and finding out the "why" might help to prevent it from happening again.

2. *Set limits.* Discuss your own values with your child and tell him explicitly what you expect of him. Listen to your child's viewpoint and try to incorporate that information into your expectations. Be sure to define what is and is not acceptable behavior. Try to be realistic in your expectations.

3. *State the consequences.* (Note: You may want to refer to the information presented in Appendix A and B.) Talk to your child about the natural consequences that could result from his behavior (for example, drug addiction, sexually transmitted disease) as well as the consequences *you* will impose if the behavior is repeated (for example, restriction of privileges, professional counseling). Ask your child to come up with an appropriate disciplinary action to fit the offense. This will increase the likelihood that he will avoid doing it again. Be clear in what you will do to prevent the behavior from becoming problematic.

4. *Follow-up.* It is important that you devise some way to follow up or monitor your child to make sure the behavior does not recur. Let your child know how you plan to follow up (i.e., what actions you will take to find out what he is doing) and how long you will do so. In the event that the behavior should happen again, remind your child of the consequences you imposed and carry them out. Back up your words with action.

A Night of Celebration

Jeff, a high school junior on the varsity football team, came home after a game smelling of alcohol. His parents confronted him about his behavior saying, "Your breath smells of alcohol. Have you been drinking?" When Jeff admitted to having three beers with his teammates, his parents asked him, "Why did you drink with them?" Jeff said that the team had just won the most important game of the season and that he had scored the winning touchdown. "The older guys were all congratulating me and offered to buy me a drink. For the first time, I really felt like one of the big shots on the team."

After getting more information about the incident, Jeff's parents were convinced that he had had almost no prior experience with alcohol and that this was a one-time incident. Jeff's father said, "I'm proud of what you did in the game, and I know how much it means to be accepted by the seniors, but you are not allowed to drink alcohol. Your mother and I won't let you drink until you are legally old enough. While you live in this house, that is the rule."

Jeff began to protest, saying that all the guys drank after the games. His parents talked to him about the problems Jeff and his friends could face if the police caught them and the possibility of injuries if they were to drink and drive. His mother said, "If we find out you've been drinking again, we will report it to your coach and take you off the football team. That may sound harsh, but we are really concerned about your safety and strongly believe you should not be drinking." Jeff's father added, "I'm sure not *all* the guys drink after the game. It's okay to turn it down. Tell your friends that getting caught means you're off the team. And whatever you do, don't get in a car when the driver has been drinking. Call us or get a ride with someone else. If you care about your friends on the team, you'll tell them not to ride with anyone who is drinking."

Jeff's parents told him that they would be checking on him after each game to make sure he was not drinking. Fortunately, Jeff got the message and never repeated the episode. His parents made it a point to meet him at the door a few times after the games to be sure, but they soon began to trust him again. Had he not obeyed the rule, Jeff's parents were prepared to follow through with their word and contact the coach.

What if the problem were bigger than that? What if Jeff continued to drink, or if his coach contacted his parents about his erratic behavior, or if he continued to show several signs of alcohol abuse? When there are many signs of a problematic behavior or when the signs persist despite interventions, it is time to acknowledge the problem and seek help.

Dealing with the Persistent Problem

Continued involvement with drugs and alcohol may indicate that your child is addicted to those substances. Dealing with an addiction or with a pattern of substance abuse cannot be successfully accomplished by parents alone. It is crucial that parents enlist the aid of qualified professionals or other resources to assess the extent of the problem and treat it.

You are not "copping out" in seeking outside help; nor are we "copping out" in recommending you do so. The hope that "he will grow out of it" is an empty one that can only lead to a steady worsening of the problem. If your child had a life-threatening disease, you would seek professional care to treat it. Substance abuse and addiction are also life-threatening and require proper treatment.

Teenage sexual activity is somewhat different in that the determination of whether or not it is problematic is partially related to one's moral, ethical, and religious beliefs. The persistence of any behavior that is expressly forbidden by parents, particularly if that behavior is flaunted or if the behavior seems uncontrollable, is, however, problematic to the family. Teens who use sexual activity to feel emotionally fulfilled or to act out angry impulses may be exhibiting signs of an emotional disorder.

It is important to seek qualified help in assessing the situation. Resources in the community are also available to counsel teens about the risks of sexual activity and how to minimize these. If a teenager is going to have sex, he or she needs to know how to take precautions to avoid pregnancy and sexually transmitted diseases, particularly in light of the current AIDS epidemic.

Seeking help from competent sources is the best way to get a realistic assessment of the severity of the problem. Unfortunately, parents often feel that seeking help is like admitting defeat. In reality, it means that they care about their child enough to set aside their own feelings of anger, disappointment, embarrassment, or helplessness to get him the help he needs.

The message here is an important one, yet too many people ignore it. Stop right now and consider it with an open mind. "But what if there really isn't a problem? I will have made a big deal over nothing." In this case you will have the reassurance you need that there is no problem, and your child will have the reassurance that you will take action if you suspect he or she is in danger. We create problems by thinking we can handle something ourselves or by waiting to make sure the problem really exists. Think of the cancer victim who wants to give the "lump" a few months to go away before "making a big deal about it" and having it examined.

The following provides a partial list of available sources, what they can do, and how to locate them:

1. *School guidance counselors.* Most schools have trained personnel on staff to assist students with career plans. Often they are trained to identify problematic behaviors and refer students to appropriate resources for help. In some cases, counselors or school psychologists are available to deal directly with the problem by offering counseling and advice. Contact your child's school to find out what it can do.

2. *Clergy.* Pastors, priests, ministers, rabbis, and other clergy are often called upon in times of family crisis to assist in counseling. Although they typically deal with the moral and ethical aspects of a particular problem, providing support and advice, many are trained to recognize and refer more serious problems for treatment. Consult your church or synagogue.

3. *Self-help groups.* These groups are for people with similar problems who meet and share advice and support about ways they have dealt with that problem. Such groups as Al-Anon, Narc-Anon, Tough Love, and others give family members help in dealing with someone who is abusing substances. These groups are listed in the phone book.

The groups listed above share the advantage of being free of charge or low cost. The disadvantage is that many people associated with these groups do not have adequate training to actively treat a persistent problem such as drug abuse, depression, or severe conduct disorders.

4. *Community agencies.* Community Mental Health Centers or other community resources such as Planned Parenthood provide professional care, often on a reduced fee or sliding scale fee basis. Personnel are trained to evaluate the problem, actively intervene, or, when necessary, refer to appropriate providers. These agencies are listed in the phone book. Because they typically receive state and/or federal funding, the quality of care they provide is routinely evaluated to insure certain standards.

5. *Private practitioners.* Professionals who deal with emotional or behavioral problems include psychiatrists, psychologists, and social workers. Many specialize in dealing with certain populations (such as adolescents or families) or certain disorders (such as substance abuse). These professionals are trained to diagnose and treat. They often work in conjunction with other agencies (hospitals, schools) to provide more individualized treatment, much like a "family doctor." They are listed in the phone book. Most large counties and all states have professional associations which can give you referrals (e.g., "County" Psychological Association, or "State" Association of Social Workers).

6. *Hospitals.* Many hospitals have programs to treat drug or alcohol abuse or other psychological problems that adolescents face. Staff are trained to diagnose and treat, and treatment often entails an inpatient stay. Hospital programs are listed in the phone book and many are advertised.

Where should you turn for help? The decision depends on many factors. If the problem seems severe or if you don't know the severity of it, it is probably best to turn to more highly trained sources who are capable of making accurate diagnoses or evaluations. *Be sure to check the credentials* of anyone who works with you or your child.

1. What kind of educational training does the person have?
2. Does that person have specialized training (for example, with substance abuse or with adolescents)?
3. Is the person licensed or credentialed by the state?
4. Has the person worked with similar problems before? If so, how many cases?

In many instances, treating an adolescent involves treating the family, and parents may be asked to participate in therapy. This does not mean that parents are "to blame" for what has happened. Rather, it is a way of looking at the situation as a family problem. No family who has ever lived with a teenage addict, or with a pregnant teenager, remains unaffected by that teenager's problem. Working together as a family helps to heal the wounds that each member has suffered so that the family as a whole, and as individuals, can continue to grow.

Many parents ask, "What if my child won't go with me for help?" Denial of a problem can be a first sign of addiction. If you truly believe there is a reason to be concerned, then treat this problem like you would any life-threatening illness by doing whatever it takes to get your child proper treatment. The various sources you contact for help will usually have suggestions about how to get your child into treatment. The most important factor is that you recognize the seriousness of the problem and that *you* actively seek treatment on your child's behalf. The rest will usually follow as you begin working with people who are experienced and skilled in dealing with such problems.

APPENDIX A
CONSEQUENCES OF DRUG USE

MARIJUANA	

Immediate
Effects

- rapid heart rate, which can cause chest pain in people who have poor blood supply to the heart
- bloodshot eyes
- dry mouth and throat
- impaired short-term memory and concentration
- impaired coordination
- slowed reaction time
- altered sense of time
- fear of losing control, which may cause panic reaction
- muscle tension
- increased appetite
- paranoid ideation

Long-term
Effects

- impaired memory
- impaired reading comprehension
- decrease in verbal and mathematical skills
- irregular menstrual cycles
- temporary loss of fertility in men and women
- premature and low-birthweight babies delivered to mothers who smoked during pregnancy
- emphysema and cancer of the lung
- "burnout"—dullness, slow movement, and inattention

Risk of   Some users develop a psychological dependence,
Dependence   finding they need greater doses to get the same ef-
               fect. Obtaining a high can become a central focus of
               a user's life. Marijuana is stored in the body's fat
               cells and can remain in the body up to 24 days.

INHALANTS

Sources   model airplane glue, nail polish remover,
               lighter and cleaning fluids, gasoline, paints,
               cookware coating agents, hair sprays, nitrous oxide
               (laughing gas), correction fluid

Immediate   • nausea
Effects   • sneezing and coughing
               • nosebleeds
               • dizziness or lightheadedness
               • euphoria
               • tiredness
               • decreased appetite
               • decreased heart and breathing rates
               • impaired judgment and coordination
               • violent behavior
               • unconsciousness
Large   • death (aspiration of vomitus while unconscious,
doses   heart failure, suffocation by displacing oxygen
                 in the lungs, depression of the central nervous
                 system)

Long-term   • permanent damage to
Effects   —central nervous system
                 —liver
                 —kidneys
                 —blood
                 —bone marrow
                 —lungs

COCAINE

Immediate Effects	• dilated pupils
	• increased blood pressure
	• raised body temperature
	• increased breathing and heart rate
	• increased alertness
	• increased energy
	• euphoria
	• depression following initial euphoria
Large doses	• confusion
	• slurred speech
	• anxiety
	• psychological problems
Long-term Effects	• restlessness
	• irritability
	• anxiety
	• sleeplessness
	• paranoia or hallucinations
	• ulceration of mucous membrane in nose
	• death (through heart or lung failure, or by fire or explosion during use of freebase)
Risk of Dependence	A strong psychological addiction occurs fairly early in the pattern of use. Cocaine becomes very dependence-producing as users begin relying on it to avoid the depression and fatigue felt while not on the drug. Use becomes a central focus of a user's lifestyle.

ALCOHOL

Sources	beer, wine, liquor
Immediate Effects	• stimulation from small doses, but depression from larger doses
	• released inhibitions

- euphoria
- reduced coordination
- increased heart rate
- muscle relaxation
- impaired visual activity
- decreased perception of pain and fatigue
- prolonged reaction time
- impaired memory and concentration
- slurred speech

High levels of blood alcohol can cause coma, death from respiratory paralysis, or death from accident.

Long-term Effects	• alcoholism • damage to liver (cirrhosis) • damage to heart • impaired kidney function • ulcerated lining of stomach • brain damage • malnutrition • loss of memory • tremors ("rum fits") • fetal alcohol syndrome in the unborn of pregnant mothers
Risk of Dependence	The effects of physical dependency are well known; the pattern of use that can lead to dependency is not, however, as well known.

NICOTINE (cigarette smoking)

Immediate Effects	• throat irritation • paralyzed cilia in bronchi • increased bronchial secretions • increased heart rate • constriction of small blood vessels • dizziness and nausea • central nervous system stimulation

Long-term   • lung cancer
Effects   • emphysema
              • chronic bronchitis
              • heart diseases
              • stroke
              • high blood pressure
              • cancer of the mouth, esophagus, throat, larynx, pancreas, and bladder
              • peptic ulcers

Risk of   Smokers suffer both psychological and physical
Dependence   addiction.

PCP (phencyclidine)

Immediate   • increased heart rate
Effects   • raised blood pressure
              • flushing and sweating
              • dizziness
Large   • numbness
doses   • increased output of adrenalin
              • convulsions
              • coma
              • death from heart and lung failure, or from ruptured blood vessels in the brain

Long-term   • memory loss
Effects   • speech difficulties
              • auditory hallucinations

APPENDIX B
CONSEQUENCES OF SEXUAL ACTIVITY

Practices
- abstinence
- hand holding
- kissing
- touching (petting) in various degrees of intimacy
- masturbation
- outercourse (sex without penetration, including oral sex)
- intercourse

Positive Consequences
- pleasure
- release of sexual tension
- intimacy with another
- loving relationship
- pleasing your partner
- procreating

Negative Consequences
- guilt
- emotional hurt
- suffering molestation or abuse
- unwanted pregnancy
- sexually transmitted diseases:
- —honeymoon cystitis, genital warts, herpes, pelvic inflammatory disease, gonorrhea, syphilis, trichomonas, yeast infection, precancerous lesions, AIDS

170

APPENDIX C

CONTRACEPTION

Note: The effectiveness rates cited are those for the "typical" user. Thus, for some methods, a method has a lower rate *not* because the method itself may fail but because the user may fail to use the method correctly.

Methods	Effectiveness	Comments (risks/benefits)
BARRIER METHODS		
• condom	90%	Relatively inexpensive method available without prescription. Encourages male participation; discrete and easy to carry; ideal for spontaneous or infrequent sex.
		Offers protection against sexually transmitted diseases; a "safe sex" practice. Greatest risk comes from noncompliance.
• diaphragm	80%	Must be fitted by a physician and used with spermicidal gel.
		Offers some protection against sexually transmitted diseases. Risks include not using the diaphragm, possible toxic shock syndrome from wearing the diaphragm too long, and recurrent urinary tract infections.

Methods	Effectiveness	Comments (risks/benefits)
• contraceptive sponge	80–90%	Needs no fitting; available without prescription. Contains spermicide. Easy to carry; ideal for spontaneous or infrequent sex.
		Offers some protection against sexually transmitted diseases. Risks include not using the sponge, possible toxic shock syndrome from wearing the sponge too long, and leaving pieces of sponge in the vaginal canal.

BIRTH CONTROL PILLS

Methods	Effectiveness	Comments (risks/benefits)
• combined pills	98%	Contain estrogen and progestin; low-dose pills are preferred.
		Safely used by young healthy women; may offer protection against some forms of gyneco-logical cancer and against pelvic inflammatory disease; decreases menstrual pain. Cardiovascular risks include stroke, heart attack, blood clots, and hypertension; risks increase with age and smoking habits.
• minipills	97.5%	Contain progestin only.
		Offers protection against pelvic inflammatory disease; decreases menstrual pain. May cause menstrual irregularities; cardio-vascular risks unknown.

Methods	Effectiveness	Comments (risks/benefits)

INTRAUTERINE
DEVICES
* IUD   95%   Inserted by physician into the uterus; no risk of noncompliance. Increased risk of pelvic inflammatory disease and perforation of uterine walls. Many have been taken off the market due to lawsuits brought by former users.

SPERMICIDES
* gels, foams, tablets, creams   80%   Often used as a back-up method. Available without prescription.

Can be messy to use; can cause irritation. Problem of non-compliance.

NATURAL
METHODS
* rhythm   75%   Abstinence during fertile days.

Higher rate of failure from non-compliance, misreading of fertile days, or irregular menstrual cycle.

* withdrawal   75%   Removal of penis from vagina before ejaculation.

Even small amount of semen deposited outside the vagina can lead to contraception.

Methods	Effectiveness	Comments (risks/benefits)
CHANCE	10%	Intercourse without use of contraception (pregnancy not intended). It is called chance for a reason.

APPENDIX D
RESOURCES

Numerous resources exist in both the areas of substance abuse and teen sexuality. Listed here are just a few of the national resources. Consult the experts in your community: school systems, Planned Parenthood affiliates, religious organizations, health care providers, local youth organizations (such as the YMCA and the YWCA), the state and local government departments.

TEEN SEXUALITY

National Council of Churches
475 Riverside Drive
New York, NY 10027

Planned Parenthood Federation of America, Inc.
810 Seventh Avenue
New York, NY 10019

Sex Information and Education Council of the United States (SIECUS)
137–155 North Franklin
Hempstead, Long Island, NY 11550

Synagogue Council of America
235 Fifth Avenue
New York, NY 10016

National Clearinghouse for Family Planning Information
Box 2225
Rockville, MD 20852

Bridging the Gap
c/o Robert A. Hatcher
69 Butler Street
Atlanta, GA 30303

SUBSTANCE ABUSE

The National Institute on Drug Abuse
Prevention Branch, Room 11A-33
5600 Fishers Lane
Rockville, MD 20857

The National Institute on Alcohol Abuse and Alcoholism
Prevention Branch, Room 16C-14
5600 Fishers Lane
Rockville, MD 20857

National Federation of Parents for Drug-Free Youth
1820 Framwell Avenue
Suite 16
Silver Spring, MD 20901

Parents Resources Institute on Drug Education (PRIDE)
Robert W. Woodruff Building
100 Edgewood Avenue
Suite 1216
Atlanta, GA 30303

Alcoholics Anonymous
Box 459
Grand Central Station
New York, NY 10163